NO HOLES BARRED

NO HOLES BARRED

A DUAL MANIFESTO OF SEXUAL EXPLORATION AND POWER

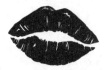

MANDII B & WEEZYWTF

WITH TEMPEST X

BLACK PRIVILEGE
PUBLISHING

ATRIA

New York   Amsterdam/Antwerp   London
Toronto   Sydney/Melbourne   New Delhi

ATRIA

An Imprint of Simon & Schuster, LLC
1230 Avenue of the Americas
New York, NY 10020

CONTENTS

TRIGGER WARNING: This book contains sensitive themes that may be emotionally challenging, including discussions related to abortion, reproductive loss, miscarriage, pregnancy loss, suicide, self-harm, sexual assault, stealthing, and victim-blaming. Chapters with these triggers are marked in the table of contents with an asterisk (*) by the title of the chapter. Please prioritize your well-being and consider skipping sections if needed. Remember, you are not alone, and support is available. Contact a trusted friend, family member, or mental health professional if you need assistance.

CONTENTS

NO HOLES BARRED

DUAL INTRO

« MANDII B + WEEZYWTF »

NO HOLES BARRED brings together our personal stories and life lessons into chapters designed to help you cultivate a healthier relationship with yourself from the inside out. As Weezy so aptly put it, "We share our fuckups so that you don't have to."

We are the sex-positive duo Mandii B and WeezyWTF. While you may not have heard of us, those who have likely know us from our podcast, *Decisions, Decisions* (formerly *WHOREible Decisions*). Vice .com described *WHOREible* as "the raciest, rawest podcast on the internet." This book delves even deeper than the pod by offering profound insights into overcoming trauma, building fulfilling relationships, and asserting control within and outside of intimate encounters.

We wanted to write a book where we could share our stories of sexual discovery, self-discovery, and growth, delivered with our signature candid, unapologetic, and always empowering attitude. We tackle complex subjects and shed light on the taboo topics most people shy away from. *No Holes Barred* is more than just a collection of experiences; it's a beacon of solidarity from us to YOU. Our goal is to empower you to live your best sexual life authentically and safely.

By sharing our individual stories, we aim to create a space where you can see yourselves reflected on the page. Maybe you'll relate more to Mandii's journey, or you might resonate more with Weezy's tales. Or you might see yourself in both of us. Regardless, we hope *No Holes Barred* serves as a mirror for those seeking to explore their sexual side while overcoming any trauma that may be holding them back.

Maybe you don't have any trauma but worry too much about what others think, allowing friends, family, and society to dictate your feelings about your sexuality. We're here to break down those barriers. While not everyone's story is the same, we hope you will see a part of yourself in this book.

No Holes Barred, like our podcast, includes real experiences and stories. However, all names are fictitious, and recognizable features have been changed. Individuals who appear in the book have given their full, willing consent. Any resemblance to others outside these permissions is purely coincidental.

No Holes Barred is designed to be a safe space. We address sensitive topics such as sexual assault, and we want you to know that chapters with these triggers are marked in the table of contents and by the title of the chapter with an asterisk (*). It's entirely up to you whether your adventure explores or skips over these sections.

At the top of each chapter, we highlight some of the **Patriarchal Bullshit** meant to keep women down. We counter those myths with **Matriarchal Replies**—empowering responses from pioneering and iconic women who have inspired us. Their voices made it possible for our podcasts to exist. These trailblazing women paved the way for a book like *No Holes Barred* to be on the shelves. We honor their legacy by dismantling the patriarchal lies and encouraging women to take ownership of their stories.

Speaking of taking the reins, after years of success with *WHOREible Decisions*, we decided to change the name of our podcast to *Decisions, Decisions*. When we chose the original name, it was a deliberate move to reclaim the word "whore" and strip it of its stigma, taking ownership of a term most often used to shame women. It felt empowering to challenge societal norms and assert our autonomy. Over time, we realized that while the name resonated with many of our fans, it also created roadblocks when working with brands and trying to expand our platform. The stigma surrounding the word "WHORE" in *WHOREible Decisions* held us back from reaching a wider audience and aligning with more mainstream brands. We're all about growing, and we see this book as integral to our evolution.

With *No Holes Barred*, we are celebrating the Power of P in a new way. This book isn't just a narrative. It's a damn revolution on how we understand and embrace our individual womanhood. Our book is deliberately divided into four transformative sections: **Pleasure, Pain, Progression,** and, ultimately, **Power.** Next we'll share our personal introductions, allowing you to get to know us better. Each of us will discuss our motivations for writing this book and explain what the Ps—**Pleasure, Pain, Progression,** and **Power**—mean to us.

Within our chapters, we share the good, the bad, the ugly, and everything in between that helped us find OUR POWER, both sexually and intimately. We've faced a lot of fear and we've broken down barriers. And ultimately, we somehow both learned to love ourselves. And trust us: if we can do it, you can, too. Our goal in writing this book is to help you find YOUR POWER.

So let our stories be a guide, a cautionary tale, and a celebration of the incredible power that lies within you. The journey to finding your power is uniquely yours, but you don't have to walk alone. We're here with you every step of the way.

INTRO

« MANDII B »

WE ENTER THIS world with very little control over the decisions made around us. We don't get to choose our family members. We don't get to choose the social class we are a part of. We don't even get to choose our names. Many of us don't recognize the impact that our upbringing has on our adulthood and, inevitably, our sexuality.

I was born into a dysfunctional, middle-class family to a white mother and a Jamaican father. The name given to me came from the mascot at what used to be Florida Hospital Orlando: Amanda the Panda. My middle name, Nicole, came from my maternal cousin's first name. And my last name was simply assigned based on the man my mother chose to get pregnant by. Everything appointed to me seemed to be secondhand and like a bit of an afterthought. I was the firstborn of what would later become known as the "house of girls." My mom, Tammi, raised me in a single-parent home with two sisters, so the presence of men was few and far between.

One weekend a month, the three of us spent time with "Daddy," who often flashed his money to try to remind us how much cooler and better he was than my mom, even though we only got to see him forty-eight hours out of the entire month. I can only recall one time when he came to see me play in any of my basketball tournaments at school. My dad was a well-paid, blue-collar construction worker who helped build water tanks for sewage waste throughout the state of Florida. Then again, as an adult, I recognize that anyone can be considered "well-paid" when they are only concerned with feeding and providing for their own damn selves. Ironically, however, cash was the only value he brought to us as a parent. Daddy was a human ATM and boasted about the very little he would contribute to our overall well-being growing up.

My mother had boyfriends, some of whom moved in, but those relationships always felt one-sided. My mother seemed to be giving more than they were, and they took whatever they wanted with little regard for how that would affect her daughters. I never referred to another man as "Dad" or viewed my mom's boyfriends as "friendly uncles" that I knew were sleeping with my mom. I watched her work multiple jobs my entire life to ensure she could support us all. At first, she waitressed at local diners and restaurants like Shoney's and Olive Garden in the evenings. Then she became a tech at the same hospital I was born in, working her way up to become a licensed practical nurse.

So here I am, the product of a failed relationship, with a front-row seat to many other failed relationships after that. There's a narrative about women growing up with "daddy issues," of course, but I don't think many of us consider the impact of relationships that we see growing up and how they will affect us on a personal level. Before we go deeper, I'd love for you to think back to the adult romantic relationships you witnessed as a child. How many of them were healthy? Which ones did you choose to ignore so that you could be what you were, a child? Did any of them become #couplegoals for you, or did you find yourself looking up to the families showcased on the Disney Channel?

Little did I know that the socioeconomic factors that impacted my family would also have a chokehold on my journey of self-exploration. To save money, my sister and I were made to share clothes and dress like twins despite being a whole year and twenty days apart. I vividly remember being teased in elementary school for wearing knockoff Adidas sneakers with four stripes instead of three. Some of our Christmas mornings were filled with presents donated from the church or the Salvation Army. We moved from one low-to-middle-income apartment to another, and life was financially and emotionally hard. It wasn't until middle school that my dad stepped in and showed off his money by getting us our first pairs of name-brand sneakers. I'll never forget—a pair of white Classic Reeboks and a black pair of K-Swiss sneakers. Foot Locker was running a two-for-$89.99 special on select styles, and I couldn't wait to sport a pair of them on the first day of school.

I remember watching movies and looking at the lives I wished I had. I'd go to my friends' homes and view what I used to think was a more "perfect" and functional family, later to find out that all that glittered wasn't gold. Much like my other friends, Weezy's life seemed the opposite of mine. I used to joke and say she was like New New, the character Lauren London plays in the movie *ATL*. While we both loved hanging with the bad boys and getting into clubs with our fake IDs, that was where the similarities ended. Weezy drove a Jaguar in high school, and her house had a perfectly manicured lawn, a huge water fountain in the front yard, and even a movie theater. The all-white home had big glass windows that allowed you to peer in and see the huge chandelier and red carpet on the stairs. Just looking inside, I imagined that the people who lived there had a life

I could only ever dream of. Her mom would always have snacks for us and be down to gossip about what was happening in pop culture or what boys we were hanging out with and entertaining. We'd leave this gated community with our drawstring ponytails and grills in our mouths, riding out to Boosie and looking like two peas in a pod. My time with Weezy and her family at her home only solidified that we lived in different worlds.

Here we are, humans placed on Earth with only one life to live. And it turns out that for the first eighteen years of our existence, we are under the supervision of people who are products of their own fucked-up circumstances. So, depending on how messed up our parents' lives were, in my mind, that dictates how difficult our child-hoods will be. I'm a '90s baby, and let's be honest: As millennials, can we say we have memories of our parents going to therapy? I can only speak for myself here, but in my primarily Black and Brown com-munity, mental health care was not an option, nor was it discussed. I'm not even going to begin to unpack how that follows us into adulthood. We have this whole book to examine that.

School was where I felt like I had the most control of my des-tiny. If I got perfect attendance, got the best grades in the class, and aced all the subjects, I would be set up to get the best job, be rich, and make a perfect wife to someone. I strove to make straight A's throughout school and even tested into the gifted program to skip second grade. My mom decided not to allow this as she wanted me to grow up around my peers. By high school, I was not only working two jobs, playing sports, and attending classes, but I began to see more of what makes life so difficult to navigate.

Friendships became more challenging to maintain as I took more responsibility for how their actions impacted my overall well-being. I began to clear the fog around my family members, who were previously given passes simply because "blood is thicker than water." I found navigating dating and showing up for people to be even more difficult than clocking in and out of my job or showing up to class on time. Why hadn't anyone explained the intricacies of human interaction to me? There should have been a class for that. Conflict resolution, forgiveness, overcoming grief, and effectively communicating emotions with people cannot be realized without the right tools.

My first job was when I was fifteen, the summer leading into tenth grade. I worked alongside my cousin at a Quiznos franchise. I made $7.25 an hour to start, and once I learned all the sandwiches, I would get a $0.25 raise. Of course, my overachieving ass learned to make all of them in the first month. I was overjoyed to finally be making my own money. When I turned sixteen, I went to work in retail at the mall and began five grueling years of folding shirts and stocking shoes. I had bills, and although it was just my cell phone and the gas to fill my 2002 Hyundai Sonata's tank, I saw how much I had to work to afford the least bit of life's joys. By this time, I had only been on a plane twice. One time, I went to St. Louis for the family reunion of one of my dad's many girlfriends, and the second time, I went to New York in seventh grade to see my half-brother off to serve in Kuwait following the 9/11 attacks. There was so much of the world for me to explore—I just knew it!

Then there were the boys. Figuring out how to start or even maintain romantic relationships with guys without a blueprint or an example of seeing a healthy relationship would prove to be a struggle. I would be remiss not to say bluntly that my thoughts on relationships were all kinds of fucked up. Call it cliché, but this was the era of *Flavor of Love,* and the height of reality television was centered around competing for love. So I figured that searching for love was a competition. Was getting a partner really any different from *The*

Hunger Games? May the strongest win—or, in many cases, the most pretty and delusional. Then, on the other end, nothing looked more fun than the lifestyle I saw the vixens living in the music videos. I wanted to lie on the big white yachts like the girls in Jay-Z's "Big Pimpin'" video and live a soft life of luxury. I would count down the days until I could be ratchet at a pool party in a thong bikini, and a man would slide a credit card down my ass crack like in Nelly's "Tip Drill" video.

By age thirteen, the idea of having a real relationship with a boy began to take shape. As I entered puberty and started dating, I became more aware of my physical appearance, which marked the beginning of insecurities about my weight and how certain parts of my body were sexualized—not just by my peers, but by adults as well. I found myself increasingly confused, struggling to understand my thoughts about my body while also grappling with how others perceived and treated me. I was supposed to be sexy, but not TOO sexy. Women were my ride-or-die friends, yet were also my direct competition in finding love. I was supposed to let a man know I liked him but then play hard to get because I couldn't come across as thirsty.

By the age of sixteen, I was fucking! Within the first year of my sexual journey, I got my cherry popped by a grade school crush, got my pussy eaten by an older woman, got pregnant by a gangbanger, and had an abortion just before going into the eleventh grade. I tapped in early on in navigating and understanding myself. I had always been physically and sexually attracted to both men and women. In recent times, more people have embraced the freedom to explore and express their sexuality in a way that feels authentic to them, using titles or labels as a means of self-expression and connection with others. This shift reflects a growing understanding and acceptance of the diverse ways in which we define ourselves.

So, for this book and to connect to many of you who have been journeying with me via the pod, I am a queer, bisexual, abrosexual, and heteroromantic cis woman. Simply put, I am very drawn to the sensuality and femininity of women; however, I only have the romantic desire to be emotionally involved with a man. While women have and will continue to join me in my physical and sexual realm, many of the moments in my life up until now were stiffly rooted in navigating a heteroromantic relationship with men. This could be partly blamed on the patriarchy, but I am still exploring what these identities mean to me.

What the fuck kinda bullshit puzzle is life? Wildly enough, being in my "Jesus Year" of thirty-three, I still feel like many of the things I pondered at thirteen are the same things I am still questioning. What is real love? Are we really all going to find our soulmates and live happily ever after? Is sex really as risky as they make it out to be? We think we will eventually get the answers to all of life's questions when, in reality, each of our experiences dictates how we receive the knowledge to make a life worth living. This journey has been so long, yet I feel like I am only scratching the surface of it all. Within this book, we're going to explore the highs and lows, the orgasms and tears, and the obstacles I overcame in finding happiness and healing.

Before I pass it over to Weezy, I want to share with you what you can expect in joining me on my journey of exploring sexuality and finding myself. I've always been exceptionally sexual and sought arousal in all forms. **Pleasure**, which presented itself naturally with the throbbing and moistness between my thighs, is the most confusing phase of this journey. People enjoy pleasure with themselves and others differently; there is no blueprint on how to achieve this. There is the internal battle of ensuring you are satisfied while navigating the external battle of society's views on what pleasure "should" be.

Then, with pleasure comes **Pain**. Pain can be a good thing, especially if you're a size queen like myself. However, there are inevitable consequences linked to sex, and without the proper channels of knowledge and/or support systems, these consequences can lead us down a path of guilt, shame, and trauma.

By far, the most important phase of our journey is **Progression**. Progression is the process of developing to a more advanced state. I would be lying to you if I told you I came into this world having all the answers. I dove headfirst into therapy when I turned thirty. I had to hold the mirror up to see how my decisions had gotten me to where I was. Why was finding true love so complicated? What was I doing to keep ending up in the same type of relationships? There were ideologies, such as accepting second place or seeking out emotionally unavailable lovers, that once made sense to me until, one day, they didn't. Reality hit me with a heartbreak and a love so intense that it led me to correct the wrong ways I'd been moving. That is how we find our **Power**. Our power comes with the strength to overcome our trauma, conquer our fears, and allow ourselves the grace to fuck up and course correct. There is a level of deprogramming that we all must do. To move into a healthier space with one's mind, body, and soul, we must hold ourselves accountable and forgive our past selves for fuckin' up. There's no right or wrong way to find yourself, but on the journey, you must set forth your intention to find and be the BEST version of yourself. I didn't always get it right. You won't, either. Buckle up as you get a front-row seat to my reality.

INTRO

« WEEZYWTF »

THE FIRST TIME I realized I was hornier than most people was around the fifth grade. I was in a computer class when I heard the AOL dial-up sound, and it was the Pavlov theory in real time. The high-pitched fuzzy buzzing as I waited for it to connect made my mouth salivate because I thought I was about to see pussy. I realized that I was different because nobody else did this. I watched the other kids' faces to see if they had also telegraphed a look of pure excitement as they wiped away their drool. But it was just me. I wiped my mouth with the back of my hand and realized I'd better get it together.

I used to find ways to hump stuff and grind on surfaces; once I got advanced, I humped my other eleven-year-old friends. I didn't have some crazy trauma that made me hypersexual or super horny. I never saw my parents have sex, had no creepy lurking uncle. I was just hyper-horny. I got to experience all of this exploration as a kid, a teenager, and an adult.

I was born in San Francisco to an Israeli father (but it's FREE PALESTINE) and a Black mother. My parents fell in love and married, showing me the ultimate example of true devotion and nurturing. My dad, Zion, owned camera shops that sold video equipment and electronics, while my mom, Jewel, a former Studio 54 party girl, was an over-the-top fabulous version of a housewife. I was lucky when it came to the freedom of sexual discussion in my home. My mom would sit around with my girlfriends and make sure we knew about our periods, how to say no to boys, and how to be safe in case we said yes. I learned about consent at the age of three. My parents would do faux scenarios about what to do if I was ever touched against my will, how to ask for help, and how to make sure that I was always in control.

Then we moved to Florida when I was about seven, and until I was fifteen years old, my life was that of an upper-middle-class kid. We had our annual vacation, we had a lovely home, we had blah, blah, blah. I don't particularly appreciate talking about this part because it tends to be a topic people like to fixate on. The fairy tale is that I had a perfect life, and when I was young, everything was handed to me on a silver platter. But that isn't the truth, and nothing is perfect. My father started losing a lot of money in the stock market while I was in high school, which shook the household. With the popularity of cell phones, why did people need to buy cameras or video cameras? My mom was constantly at the pawnshop. I remember finding the prom dress I wanted and her asking them to hold her wedding ring as collateral, and that's when it hit me. My life was changing.

In high school, I was openly and publicly hornier than most, and everyone seemed to think it was wrong. I sat around with my girlfriends to show them some of the latest porn I was watching, how we could talk with guys in chat rooms, and the next day at school, everyone called me a slut. Our friends are supposed to be our safe space, right? Maybe they could've been if it weren't for the patriarchy. They were consumed by the idea that women weren't supposed to be watching things like that, putting their minds in dirty places, and having open conversations about SEX *SEX* SEX!

After getting out of an abusive relationship, which I will share more about in chapter ten, I started my journey in the workforce at around twenty. I got a job at White House Black Market, a retail store that sells women's clothing. After a year working at this store, a client offered me a position at T-Mobile. I was living life, traveling the globe, and able to take care of my twenty-two-year-old self and my friends! I was always the one with the nice apartment, buying drinks for the crew when we were out, and it felt empowering to have my financial freedom after such a terrible relationship.

My high didn't last long; during my first real lesbian relationship, with a woman I called Scissors, my father had a stroke and became unable to work.

My mom got her first job at a clothing store to help with bills, and by the time I was twenty-three, I had become the adult responsible for my family. I managed everything from my parents' social security to rent to doctors' appointments. Frankly, this is why I grew tired of the notion that I had been some spoiled rich kid; in reality, my parents became my children, and this has been my life for over a decade.

I needed more income, so I took on a few sugar daddies. No one was more important than HIM. He had the planes, the homes, and the cold, hard cash he'd put in my hand after nights of doing nothing more than cuddling. Finally, after realizing that Orlando wasn't the place for me, I decided to move up within the T-Mobile Company to New York City. I went from an in-store sales associate to a sales executive at the corporate headquarters. He told me we could be "roommates" whenever he wanted to visit. He got me my first apartment on 54th Street and 8th Ave, a two-bedroom luxury penthouse in the sky with a doorman with gloves, and I was living my best *Sex and the City* life!

I may have been a sugar baby, but I continued to climb the corporate ladder, busting my ass in sales. I would never be wholly financially dependent on a man again. I was in the top tier for sales in my region as the youngest person to hold that position. I was also the only Black one, the only woman, and the only employee with no college degree to be selling at that level.

While in NYC, I received a message from Mandii, an old friend from Orlando who had also moved to the city and wanted to catch up. We had some drinks in the Meatpacking District, caught up about our roles in corporate America, shared some hoe stories, and by the end of it . . . we had a podcast. I devised the pun *WHOREible*, and she lengthened it with *Decisions*. We talked about our favorite podcasts and what made them special; a week later, we were in the studio for the "Missing Condom" episode. Through sharing our personal stories and sexcapades, we made a connection with our fans that became so strong there was no more time for our day jobs.

We went from doing things independently to managing teams and agents and screening people begging to be our interns. With the help of Charlamagne Tha God, we became part of iHeartMedia's Black Effect Podcast Network. Today, after millions of listening hours, performing in front of thousands of people over the years, and being covered in TV shows and magazines, we are still actively doing our podcast. I sold my first TV show, *$ex Sells*, to Fuse. My growing experience in production led me to the ears of award-winning writer Kenya Barris, who hired me as the head of his podcast division.

I have completely surpassed my wildest dreams of what my life would look like. This book is happening because what Mandii and I have created together did not exist before. We weren't necessarily sex pioneers, but we broke so many barriers for Black women through sharing our own lives on air that it only made sense to expand our reach. The story about the time a guy wouldn't take off the blindfold until his dick was in me deserves to be in more places.

I think our show is so popular because, sure, there's Google, but we NEED that crazy hoe friend to fill in the gaps when we're confused about words like "bukkake," "cuckolding," or "snowballing." If you don't have that person in your life, here we are. I want this book to be your entryway. I want to spill my secrets to you. I want to tell you all about how I was in a throuple, how I've been dominated, how I've learned to accept my kinks, even the one about blood, so you can learn to accept yours. I want this book to be a piece of your self-discovery, no matter where you are. These pages are a tribute to adult sexual education, exploration, and a lotta smut.

In the **Pleasure** section of this book, I will talk to you about the fact that pleasure isn't given; it's earned. Asking for what you want is essential. Exploration and letting go of whatever insecurities we have can lead to a better sex life. In the **Pain** chapters, I share the trauma that I've carried for over a decade. Through my conversations within the sex education community, it dawned on me that my experiences are not just my own. They are my neighbors', friends', mother's, and even yours. Sharing the pain I've been through, whether heartbreak or assault, will show you that you are not alone. The amazing part of the pain for me is that I have been able to reclaim myself and grow despite it or even because of it.

I have come to realize, especially being in my thirties, that many of the decisions I have made were based on preconceived notions regarding the outcome. I talk about this in the **Progression** section. For example, I would stay in a relationship just so someone wouldn't say, "She can never keep a man." But the actual reality was that they'd think, "Good for her for choosing herself!" I made many of my choices because I did not want to be judged by others. I don't believe we can progress without feeling disappointed by people's reactions and then finally deciding to choose ourselves. There really IS an art to not giving a fuck.

After reaching **Power**, I hope that when you finish reading this book, you will come to realize that life is short and the sex life that you desire is in your own hands (literally). There's no reason to wait for the best orgasms of your life to arrive at your doorstep. You've gotta give them to yourself, and you have to teach your partners. You are the key to your pleasure in the bedroom, the boardroom, and beyond. This book is an ode to sexual and self-exploration.

Lastly, a little bit about the personality and current life of the person who just told you all her trauma before she shared her favorite color. (It's black.)

I am passionate about life, learning, kindness, and all things Beyoncé, gastronomy, and music. In my free time, I explore new music and art, and love on my dog, Nina, in the Lower East Side of New York City.

NO HOLES
BARRED

PLEASURE

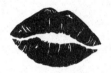

The pursuit of pleasure is the basis for much of our human experience.

By exploring our desires and letting go of insecurities,
we can create a more fulfilling sex life. Whether physical,
emotional, or intellectual, pleasure requires openness,
honest communication, and vulnerability. When we embrace this
and confidently express our needs, we open ourselves
to more profound and rewarding experiences.

You only live once, so you may as well enjoy the hell out of it!

Patriarchal Bullshit
"The sexual life of adult women
is a dark continent for psychology."
—Sigmund Freud (founder of psychoanalysis)[1]

Matriarchal Reply
"If any female feels she needs anything beyond herself
to legitimate and validate her existence,
she is already giving away her power
to be self-defining, her agency."
—bell hooks (author of *Feminism Is for
Everybody: Passionate Politics*)[2]

HOW CAN I EXPECT YOU TO PLEASE ME IF I CAN'T PLEASE MYSELF?

« MANDII B »

THE TITLE OF this chapter is a loaded fucking question. One that I've worked to try to figure out for a long time. Self-fulfillment is something that we talk a lot about in our society in a very superficial way—#selfcare. But many of us don't realize that getting to know ourselves and our bodies, and what we actually want, takes work. In this chapter I wanted to discuss achieving pleasure with yourself before acknowledging how someone else can assist you with feeling satisfied. I thought that this was going to be easy to write and that I would bang this chapter out (literally), but the further I got into it, the more I realized that my relationship with masturbation bleeds into my relationships with my partners, my views on sex, and, inevitably, myself.

According to an article on PleasureBetter.com, "women most often have their first orgasm through masturbation."[3] This was not the case for me; I didn't orgasm until after I started having heterosexual penetrative sex. So, from the beginning, I tied the idea of my pleasure to men, and it was not until the past couple of years or so that masturbating alone became completely fulfilling to me. This shift happened because at some point, without even knowing it, I let go of my sexual power. And recently, I learned how to snatch that shit back. But for me to get to this place, it took time, growth, and self-reflection through therapy.

My issues with my lack of self-worth started where they do for many of us: in my childhood, back when I was young and impressionable. There are a myriad of layers that impacted my early views of self. I can admit to my "daddy issues" and could place the blame on him for not being present enough. I could add being pissed at my mom for working so much and not telling me not to seek validation from men like she did. I watched my mom constantly fall into relationships with men who didn't deserve her love and who took advantage of her kindness. I wish she would've shared those lessons with my sisters and me in the moments she felt exploited. It was also not the easiest experience being slut-shamed by my teachers throughout grade school simply because my hips, thighs, and breasts developed early and my body was that of a grown woman. I found puberty to be tough as I dealt with my "grown woman weight." I felt uncomfortable in my own skin, all while getting an overwhelming amount of unwanted attention from the boys in school and grown-ass men who had no business looking in my direction. I didn't have a father figure to talk to me about all the ways men show up as tricksters to get what they want out of women.

However, if I'm being honest, when I was young, there were times when my pleasure was all mine, even if the experiences did not end with a big (or even a little) O. I am going to start at the beginning and tell you about the first times I remember feeling that rush. The heat. The heartbeat thumping between my legs. When I was little, I remember being very clear about who I was and striving to know what I liked and disliked. I knew what my favorite television shows were, which foods I preferred over others, and what music resonated with me. I was eager to be just as sure and clear about the things I liked and disliked when it came to my body, my pleasure, and how I wanted to feel. I felt that sensation for the first time with a giant teddy bear. Yes! You read that right.

My parents had a tumultuous relationship, to say the least. I was five years old when my mom decided she'd had enough of my dad's shit. She packed up the basics, took my sister and me, and moved us from the Americana apartment complex to a town house at Ashley Point. Now, mind you, our new place was within walking distance of the old one. When my mom left my dad, she never ran very far away. Eventually, Daddy would storm into the next place and take charge like he was the king. That was the cycle. He had very little regard for my mom's feelings or the relationships she chose to move on to after theirs. I know this shaped my views on dating—but only the negatives. I knew exactly what I *didn't* want, but I never had an example of a healthy relationship.

Because Mommy had left Daddy, we had very little money. She was working as a waitress, so we were surviving on the tips she made. That Christmas, we were blessed because a lot of people from our church went out of their way to help us get stuff for the new house. My favorite gift that year was a gigantic Christmas bear from my granny. He was a light-caramel overstuffed bear about three feet tall with a festive red bowtie. I slept with him for a long time. I'm unsure when I started hopping on top of Christmas Bear and rubbing my crotch on him for pleasure, but it wasn't too long after. The friction created this heated sensation between my legs, and, well, I loved it. I liked the heat. A lot. And, of course, I thought, *What the fuck is happening?* But I also thought, *This feels good.* And that was enough.

As an adult, I know that when I say I was only five, that sounds young. But after doing some research, many kids start exploring their bodies between the ages of three and five, so I was right on time. When I got to third grade, I found a replacement for Christmas Bear. I discovered the detachable showerhead. My mom says we'd always had them, but I guess I could finally reach it and take it down myself. The vibration and how the water made my erogenous zones light up was magic. My mom had no idea what I was using that goddamn showerhead to do. I was young, and once again, my pleasure was still all mine.

I met my friend, we'll call her Amber, on the first day of kindergarten. Our teacher, Miss McDonald, announced it was finally time for our parents to leave. This tiny girl in a ruffled quinceañera-looking dress started to melt down. As the confident kid that I was, feeling bad for her, I immediately went over to comfort her. From that day on, Amber and I were always together. My mom became a tech at the hospital and started attending nursing school to get her nursing license, so I spent most of my weekends at Amber's house.

At some point, when I was sleeping over, Amber and I started playing "the game." It's weird. We never talked about it or questioned it. We wouldn't even plan it. We would just be like, "Let's play 'the game.' Right? Okay. Let's play!" And so, we would begin hunchin' and kissing each other on her little wooden bed.

According to *Youth Today*, common behaviors of children from six to twelve years old include "experimentation with same-age children, often during games, kissing, touching, exhibitionism and role-playing."[4]

Today, my friend Amber is not bisexual or gay. And I am absolutely bisexual. It is natural for us to explore our sexuality throughout different times in our lives. For parents and caregivers reading this, I would encourage you to be open to your children doing the same as you did. Whether you hunched your friend during slumber parties or found yourself in a relationship with a stuffed animal, you're aware of the natural progression of your own sexual exploration.

I started devouring all the erotica books that I could get my hands on around fifth grade. I tore through *Addicted* and the *Chocolate Flava* series by Zane. I loved *Pleasure* by Eric Jerome Dickey. I can't go through Black erotica books without mentioning my absolute favorite: Sister Souljah's *The Coldest Winter Ever*. My mom was so happy when I asked for a book for Christmas one year that she didn't even bother to inquire about what filth and drama I was filling my little brain with. Even though I wasn't having all the sex that Winter was, I was hardheaded like Winter and a natural-born hustler. I couldn't get over reading erotica and how it made my body feel.

I also found myself indulging in celebrity fan fiction message boards. You know the ones, right? While reading erotic fan-fiction stories, I could imagine myself fucking my favorite stars. B2K was a popular urban boy band in the early 2000s. As I read the message boards (which you can still find today—I know 'cause I looked), I'd imagine that Lil' Fizz and J-Boog were both doing nasty things to me at the same time while I dated their "homeboy" Bow Wow; I devoured stories about having sex with Chris Brown while Lloyd walks into the room and joins in. Why TF was I thirteen years old and being turned on by the thought of being in a fucking GANG-BANG? I'm literally laughing thinking back about how I was born to be a freak because I loved this shit!

I felt like my heartbeat was in my pussy while I read these tales. I'd feel a thump-thump-thump down there. And I was like, *Oh, I like this*. I would sneak onto the desktop computer in the house late at night and pray the dial-up noise didn't wake anyone. I'd be glued to the screen, reading the filthiest narratives while nature took its course between my thighs. I just knew I wanted that electric feeling. Things had accelerated from a heated sensation to thumping to a full-blown puddle of wetness. And though my mind had been hard at work helping me reach arousal, I still didn't know how to masturbate and orgasm. I would just sit in the puddle, feeling my pussy throb, and enjoy this rush of excitement and pleasure.

Though it may sound strange that I did not know how to cum, it is actually the norm. According to Adam & Eve, it turns out that "if you're like most women, you probably experienced that blissful moment somewhere between the ages of 18 to 24 . . . which conducted a survey that found 45 percent of women crossed the finish line for the first time during that age range. Coming in at a close second, 43 percent of women said they took their first trip to O-town before their 18th birthday."[5]

As I mentioned earlier, my body developed at a rapid rate and my curves arrived earlier than they did for many of my peers. I remember being on the morning announcements in the fifth grade and folding my arms high in front of me so the boys wouldn't make mention of my cleavage. Even in middle school, the boys differentiated me as "Amanda with the Big Butt." My teachers and basketball coaches sexualized me and accused me of being fast even though I hadn't even had my first kiss. I found myself being lectured by my teachers about the time I would spend around boys, and the conversations would always lead to why it was so important to stay a virgin. I was being sexualized by my peers and grown-ass fuckin' adults at every turn. I remember feeling guilty of God knows what and ashamed of myself when I hadn't done anything wrong. Apparently, where I was in Florida, if you had hips, it was because they'd spread from fucking and were ready for childbearing. How fuckin' stupid!

My mom had to cuss out the school all the time because they would accuse me of dressing inappropriately while the girls who were much smaller were wearing skirts infinitely shorter than mine. Being sexualized by hella adults made me want to prove everyone wrong. I was going to show them I wasn't who they believed I was by simply not doing anything. I wanted to steer as far from boys and sex as possible. By middle school, I was far behind my friends. I remember thinking, *Y'all worried about the wrong bitch. My friends are the ones! Yeah, tiny hips over there is the girl who's already getting it.* Other people stepped in and made me feel some way about myself. I felt like pleasure, or even the idea of it, was a bad thing and would attach a negative stigma to me.

I stayed a virgin through my first year of high school when I began to feel peer pressure. I was the last virgin out of all my friends, and a part of me felt left out. When I finally did lose my virginity, it was to my schoolgirl crush. The sex was not very memorable, but the person I lost it to? His beauty was unparalleled. I had skipped many steps here. I hadn't even navigated my own pussy before I gave it up to an inexperienced teenage boy. This was the beginning of leaving my pleasure up to someone else.

By the time I was in my junior and senior years, I was dealing with men; by my last year of high school I was being flown out by an

NBA player obsessed with making me squirt. Yes, squirt! Like many women, I was finally able to climax at the age of eighteen because he was the first person to make me cum. I had definitely enjoyed sex with different people, but he was the first man focused on my pleasure and making me cum more times than himself.

When we first met, he was twenty-one. He'd just graduated college and gone into the league. He was 6'10", with a medium chocolate complexion and braids he was ready to loc. We had quite a few mutual friends and ended up meeting on Facebook. Before going to the league, he went back to Atlanta where he was from. We began seeing each other early mornings, and I was fucking him crazy before he'd drop me off at school in his white Porsche Cayenne. We ended up moving back to Orlando from Atlanta at the end of my junior year, and I was sure I would never see him again. But I was wrong. By the time I was eighteen, he was in his second year playing in the league. I was still in my senior year, and he was playing in California. Visiting him would end up being my first trip to the West Coast and my very first time going into a sex store.

This is the moment when his desires transformed into what I convinced myself I wanted, blurring the line between his aspirations and my own needs. I ultimately allowed him to take the lead in our sexual experiments. I was curious and eager to try new things and test the boundaries of my body. I trusted him in the bedroom, and I was open to allowing him access to all of my holes and beyond for research purposes. HE already had a plan for what he wanted to do with me because he'd been watching videos of women squirting and wanted me to do just that. HE was enamored with being able to hold power over a woman and make her scream and orgasm with her visibly cumming. I say "visibly cumming" because, for many women, our orgasms happen on the inside of our walls, and we don't usually get the fun cum shot that men have when they orgasm. HE took me to my first sex shop and bought a bunch of toys and this massive wand that had to be plugged into the wall. It vibrated at speeds I had never felt, and I was a bit intimidated, feeling like it would be used as a jackhammer on my poor lil' clit. I remember him reassuring me that this specific toy was the key to helping me achieve HIS squirting goal. HE told me that this was going to feel incredible for me. And here I was thinking, *How does he know? Has this nigga's pussy ever squirted before?*

I'd never even used a toy, and the vibration was a lot—it was too damn much. My mind wouldn't let me relax. There was no way I was going to squirt. No squirting came from this experiment. It didn't happen the time after that, either. Or the next time. But HE was on a mission. And almost a whole year later, HE finally made me squirt. HE found the spot with his hands. And boy, did it feel amazing. I cried after the release. But at what cost? Because by this time, the relationship was toxic as fuck.

It was toxic the way we argued constantly, and we only found ourselves enjoying each other in the bedroom. In the bedroom, we were in love. Outside of the bed, I hated this motherfucker with a passion. Our personalities did not mesh at all. He had a short temper and could not express himself in a way that didn't come off as combative. I also hated how many video games he played in his free time and how he was ill-equipped to navigate his grief from a lot of loss at an early age. I remember him introducing me to his teammate as his "friend," which allowed me backdoor advancements. I ended up sleeping with his teammate, and when he confronted me about it, I told him that we were only "friends" and that I could talk to whoever I wanted. Despite being upset by my actions, we couldn't get enough of each other. Because the sex was that good, for a long time, HE was the only one I could squirt with. I thought that HE held the power over my body and my pleasure. Not me. It didn't matter what shitty things he said to me or how bad he'd make me feel. I'd keep him around and continue seeing him to feel that rush and feeling he brought me. Just because he's good for your hole doesn't mean he's good for your soul. Remember that.

Exactly two days after graduating high school, I packed up my Hyundai Sonata and moved back to Atlanta. I got myself a cute little apartment. I was eighteen years old and ready to explore without the boundaries of living under my mom's roof. The world was mine, and boy, did the freedom of having an apartment make it easy to get laid. I lived with a girl about five years my senior, and she introduced me to all the things. I had met her through a mutual friend, and we were both looking for a place at the same time. Living with her got pretty wild. I remember, at one point, she would invite me into her room to watch her suck one of her many lovers. Eventually, we would tag team them, and I'd join in entirely. We even both shared a cute, tatted dread head who lived down the hall.

By this time, I thought I was "that" bitch. I had morphed into the kind of woman Sister Souljah would write about in her books. It was a lot of sex without the drugs, drama, and murders. But the ironic thing was, like many women in her books, I found myself deeply depressed. I'd call my mom spiraling because if I went two or three weeks without sex, I felt like I was going to pull my hair out. My mom, of course, had no idea how to help me cope with my thoughts at the time. We never had the birds and bees conversation; she only found out I was having sex when I came to her pregnant. My dry spells from sex would lead me to extremes, and at one point, I even thought I would literally kill myself if I didn't have sex. I had become so reliant on my sexual worth being connected to other people that I didn't feel comfortable just by myself.

I was masturbating a lot and, finally, to completion by the time I reached my early twenties. Having that hot rush of release instead of just feeling the tension was fucking incredible. Learning what I liked alone became about testing things I might want to try with others. I would talk to myself and realized that it made me wetter. Aha moment! I should tell my partner to be more verbal. I realized I enjoyed massaging my clit in slow circular motions. So the next time I was getting head and they wanted to be Speedy Gonzales on my pearl, I knew to tell them to slow it down. There were moments during self-pleasure when I would squeeze my breast. I found myself moving my lover's hands over my body the same way in which I would. Nonetheless, I had not found a way to find pleasure from penetrating my hole through all of this. These T-Rex arms were too short to enjoyably penetrate my pussy without an inanimate object.

That was the problem. I needed that dick, and at the same time, I realized that sex became about having another person to validate my need to be desired. There is nothing wrong with wanting to be wanted. However, it's another thing when someone else's view of you defines your self-worth.

Do you know how you and your girls used to really think that a guy would love you and want you more when you gave him some pussy? Boy, who the hell told any of us this?

I'd yo-yo between thinking my vagina was just the best, that my juicy pussy was all that any man could ever want, and being let down time and time again. Because giving it to them did not make them stay. During this period, my weight also fluctuated drastically, and I was super insecure about it. I was surviving off bartending tips like my mother once had and struggled financially as I moved from Atlanta to Miami to finally end up in New York by the age of twenty-two. I'd wallow in the thoughts of what I envisioned my life should be compared to the reality of the survival mode I found myself in. I couldn't even recognize myself anymore. I spent years like this, forgetting what I liked and how to please myself.

And then the best thing happened to me. I went through a traumatic breakup at thirty-two. Yes, bitch, my first heartbreak was at the big-ass age of thirty-two. This man shattered my fucking heart into a million little shards. I had experienced my first heartbreak, and somehow, that shit led me to find more of myself in a way I would have never imagined. I was so broken that I finally accepted that I needed to figure out the root of why I continued to be in these unhealthy relationships with men specifically. I was rocked to my foundation. Shaken to my core. I could fall into the hole or rebuild. I finally saw that the validation I so desperately sought outside of myself was just a Band-Aid over something I had yet to face.

So I decided to rebuild and to get help. Because this was something I realized I could not fix on my own, I did something incredibly difficult for me: I asked other people for help. I started by working with an incredible therapist. I began to have open and authentic conversations with the people I trusted who were willing to aid me in my healing. I used the access that I have to sexual health experts from doing the podcast, and I learned from them. And probably the most critical decision I made was to stay single and abstain from sex. Instead of hopping right into another relationship or even a situationship, I decided to work only on my relationship with myself. Well, to be honest, I did initially hop back onto a dick that was for sure going to make me feel better. However, it didn't. I remember feeling utterly empty after we fucked, and disgusted with myself. I needed a break from men and sex.

This is when I finally had that moment of clarity and realized that THEY couldn't give me what I needed. Only I had the real power to do that. It sounds cliché as fuck, but learning to love me is the only thing that can fill me up. I took a year off from dating and went through bouts of no sex during this time. I still needed pleasure because I'm a sexual fucking being, but I achieved it by myself. The more I have learned to love myself, the more I have found pleasure in playing by myself. I no longer seek an outside source to give me what I need. I can give it to myself.

The thump-thump-thump is now the sound of my heart pounding after I've cum, before I fall asleep, alone and satisfied. Because the next time I let anyone near my body, it is going to have to be about true intimacy and a connection I can't get within myself. Until then, I got me.

MASTURBATION FACTS & TIPS

Exploring self-pleasure is essential in understanding your sexual preferences. It allows you to discover your preferred touch, pressure, and rhythm. Mastering self-pleasure can facilitate better communication with your partner about what brings you satisfaction. Being confident in your sexual experiences and communication makes it easier to prioritize protection against STDs and unintended pregnancy.

Research has shown the health benefits of masturbation. Masturbation can:

- Release sexual tension
- Reduce stress
- Help you sleep better
- Improve your self-esteem and body image
- Relieve menstrual cramps and muscle tension

I want to share some tips that help me reach an orgasmic climax when I'm by myself.

BE INTENTIONAL ABOUT ALONE TIME—Many struggle to find time and space for themselves. Whether you're a parent, live with a significant other, or share your living space with roommates, it can seem like pleasuring yourself is impossible because others are around. However, it's essential to set aside time just for you. Maybe it's when the kids are at school, your partner is at the gym, or your roommate is at work. Make sure you carve out those moments where you have the freedom to enjoy your own company.

SET THE MOOD—If you enjoy sex with a specific playlist or ambiance when you're with someone else, create that same atmosphere when you're alone. You can even make a playlist specifically for your solo time. Also, ensure your space is clean and comfortable. Light candles, wear something that makes you feel good, and create an environment to relax and enjoy the experience.

MOAN—This might sound a little silly, but it works! The same sounds you make when you're with someone else can enhance your experience when you're by yourself. Moaning out of pleasure can intensify the moment, and sometimes, the louder I moan, the better my orgasm feels.

ENGAGE YOUR SENSES—To become more comfortable with your body and truly enjoy self-pleasure, it's important to explore your senses. While touching yourself, take moments to bring your fingers to your nose and become familiar with your scent. As you get more aroused, taste yourself. Embrace the sensations and appreciate the natural essence your partner experiences when they enjoy you.

I'd like to preface this chapter by letting you know that
I masturbated midway through writing page 29
because the details are just . . . HOT!

You're welcome, reader.

Patriarchal Bullshit
"I like threesomes with two women, not
because I'm a cynical sexual predator. Oh no!
But because I'm a romantic. I'm looking for 'The One.'
And I'll find her more quickly if I audition two at a time."
—Russell Brand (English comedian, actor,
presenter, activist, and campaigner)[1]

Matriarchal Reply
"Maybe we were never meant to do it with
only one other person. Maybe threesomes were
the relationship of the future."
—Carrie (Sarah Jessica Parker's character
on *Sex and the City*)[2]

WHY DON'T WE CHEAT TOGETHER?

« WEEZYWTF »

CAN YOU CARE about someone else so much that their pleasure becomes yours? Not just in ways that are easily accessible but in ways that society will judge us for—hell, ways that we may even judge ourselves for. I don't know when my brain started to go left instead of right, but at some point I became extremely attracted to the thought of watching my partner with someone else.

I grew up with a mother who loved being a housewife, which greatly influenced my idea of what a family should look like. My parents were a "normal" hetero-monogamous couple. While my mother desired and loved being a "domestic engineer" and not working outside the home, this wasn't my dream or the ideal for many women in America. However, the patriarchy would have us thinkin' something different.

Mainstream media example of the patriarchy as seen on my TV:

Virginal young woman meets a man with more experience. Man chooses young woman. They get married. Monogamy. Cookie-cutter wife. Monogamy. Husband goes to work. Monogamy. One boy. Monogamy. One girl. Wife cooks. Wife cleans. Wife runs errands. Church. Monogamy. Monogamy. Monogamy. Monogamy. White picket fence. More monogamy. THE END.

I didn't necessarily have an issue with what I saw on television, and it was homogeneous with my mother's advice about how to keep a man. When I became a teenager and started dating, we had intense conversations about how to "KEEP YOUR FUTURE HUSBAND HAPPY," which was basically that he wouldn't be led astray by some new pussy if I kept a perfect home and did acrobatics in the bedroom. Not that it was anyone's fault, but I was brainwashed into believing that love meant you didn't cheat. But does the appeal of another sexual partner really mean that our spouse doesn't love us? Cheating to me means there is downright lying or deceit going on.

But I've come to learn that the idea of "cheating together" is probably going to be my thing! I guess the thought of watching has always turned me on, so maybe my younger self knew I was different. I think it was the older version of me who needed to catch up—the version that was judged and told that this shit ain't normal, and this isn't the kind of thing that I should want. But I do enjoy it. And that's all that matters to me at this point in my life.

I've had threesomes, which I enjoyed, but I often wondered about how I liked to participate in them. How come I would stop sucking dick for a second just to look? Why would I fake an orgasm so that my turn would be over and I could lean back and take in my partner fucking someone else? My active participation in the threesome was not always the point; it was to *watch*.

Now, mind you (Black-ass thing to say, by the way), I had no real conscious idea about what I was doing when I was doing it. I thought that maybe I liked watching because it felt like live porn. I couldn't figure it out.

Sometimes, I'd have threesomes with my own partner, but it would always be on my terms. Now, maybe it's the ego in me, needing to know that even though my partner was with someone else, it was "just sex" and there was more than that with me. That we fucked someone else, yes, but we were the two people who had a real connection. We had a depth between us that the person joining us was not a part of and could never comprehend. I wanted all of us to get off and have a good time together, but I wanted to know that my partner was uniquely mine.

With one partner, I often didn't feel as excited as I thought I should, but the idea of us getting off together with a third used to get me going like nothing else . . . that is, until it became less about me and more about my partner and the third party. Maybe it's a part of my submissiveness. Who knows?

What I do know is that it truly started with Scissors . . .

But the reality is that it was *compersion.*

The word "compersion" refers to finding joy in the joy of others. In the world of consensually non-monogamous relationships, it relates to the happiness someone derives from their partner seeking out and enjoying sexual and romantic intimacy with other people. I experience true pleasure while watching someone I care about receive pleasure. It's almost like this game in my head where I feel power and security in handling their exchange with someone else.

The most significant difficulty I've had in accepting this weird-ass kink is that other people don't believe me. It's a constant insecurity I face since I have been vocal about the fact that I'm looking for a committed relationship and love. Other people say, "HoW yoU

GoN sAY yOU Don'T wANnA gEt CHeATEd ON bUt yOU oPeNinG pAndoRa'S boX?"

Do these people who judge my life not think I could want the things I engage in? I continually hear from others that a man is taking advantage of me, that he is why "I think" I want these things. But I can easily dismiss that thought. Because when the first feelings of compersion happened to me, it wasn't about a man. It all started with her. Her fulfillment also became mine.

Scissors is the nickname of my ex-girlfriend. I still believe she and I had one of the healthiest relationships I've ever been in. Our relationship was a long-distance one from the start. Well, the third start . . . more on that later. Scissors lived in Florida, and I lived in New York. By the third time we got together, Scissors knew I was truly a bisexual woman. When I look back on it now, I really hope she never considered my craving for men to mean that I didn't want her or that she didn't make me happy. It's just that sometimes, I like to switch up the menu a little!

We had known each other from high school and being on the scene in Orlando, where we became friends and eventually lovers. We weaved in and out of dating while spending time together, and ironically only entered a serious relationship once I had moved out of Orlando. I called Scissors to hang out when I came back for Thanksgiving, and we went dancing with friends. That night, I started to flirt with a fan I ran into in the club, and to my surprise, Scissors got jealous. She went off on me in the bathroom, a fight that turned into a make out that turned into sex, and made me late to Thanksgiving dinner the next day. My reconnection with her at twenty-six made me realize she was someone I didn't want to be without. Our communication intensified after this trip, and the reconnection became a long-distance relationship.

Since we were living in different states, we had this unspoken understanding about our sexual needs outside of each other. We never had a full-blown conversation about boundaries at the time since we both were inexperienced, but we found ways to enjoy the time apart. While away, we'd get someone's number on a night out with friends—we might even use those digits and fuck the person— but I was never trippin' because I knew where home was. And she didn't trip, either, because she felt the same way. We both told each other everything. That was part of what made our partnership so special. We didn't hide our cravings from one another. We shared them with each other. And it was also part of what made our part- nership so fucking hot! I couldn't wait to share my kinky stories with her, and I also loved to hear all the sordid details of her time with other people.

One day, after having a particularly fun night with a partner named "Beard Bae," I called Scissors and told her the juicy details of my latest encounter. She was really into it. In the past, we had always tossed the idea around of having a threesome, but frankly, what couple hasn't?

Over the years of doing our show, Mandii and I have joked about how many emails we get from couples with questions about three- somes. You all are out there doing a lot of daydreaming. But we are glad that you share with us because that is a hell of a lot healthier than doing the opposite and going for it without thinking it through.

Some people never consider the "what ifs."

What if you get into a threesome and your partner is intensely making out with the other person? What if you don't like how that makes you feel? What if they are overcomplimentary of the third? "Damn, your body is so fucking amazing." But they've never said shit like that to you, or maybe not in a long-ass time. What if they have a fast orgasm with the new person because it is just so damn good? What if they scream louder, cum harder?

Still in it? Will you still feel like this is something you want?

Well, I'm the girl who knows she likes it. Scratch that. I LOVE IT. Jealousy can truly be hot. Hear me out.

A relationship is a constant game of trying not to disappoint each other; involving other people can clearly put that at risk. Unequivocal trust is the foundation for having a successful three-way relationship. It's a good idea to explore the possibilities of the worst and best that can happen. There are many questions to ask yourself before knowing if a third would enhance your relationship, but in this instance, I'll narrow it down to three.

1. Would watching your partner receive affection from or give affection to someone else turn you on?

2. Do you feel more excited than anxious by the idea of fulfilling this sexual fantasy?

3. Does your partner have enough emotional maturity and healthy communication skills to deal with feelings that may arise in the aftermath?

If your answer to these three questions is YES, GET READY FOR SOME FUN.

Scissors and I agreed that having a threesome with a man was something that we both wanted to do. After consenting and confirming with Scissors that Beard Bae, whom she had only heard stories about but never met, would be a viable option for our first go at a threesome, I called him up. I started the convo off slowly with some light small talk. I could tell Beard Bae was ready to get off the phone, so I laid it on him.

Me: Okay, well . . . I kinda have something I need to ask you.

BB: Well, what is it?

{Super Awkward Silence}

BB: I gotta go. So . . .

Me: I don't want you to feel like you're obliged to say yes. I really want you to take your time to think this through.

BB: Nigga, spit it out!

Me: Okay, so I've been talking with Scissors, and we were thinki—

BB: YES! OH MY FUCKING GOD, WEEZY. I BEEN WAITING FOR YOU TO ASK ME THIS SHIT.

And then I started our group chat TREYWAY.

Now, I won't act like ya girl is some manipulative mastermind, but I know a thing or two about women. The main thing I know is that within a threesome dynamic, the primary partners must never feel threatened by the third. Being that I'd had sex with Beard Bae before and Scissors knew it, I wanted to make sure that she felt comfortable and not left out. I started talking about my previous sexual experiences with him like I'd test-trialed the dick for her. I acted like I'd done us both a favor to make sure that dick was good enough before she had it. Maybe I am a bit of a sexual mastermind . . .

The night started with us meeting up at Story Nightclub. We got in at 1 a.m. The place was totally packed. Crazy. Typical Miami shit. Bodies upon bodies upon bodies crammed together. The bottle girls, who only smile at you if you're with the biggest baller in there, were pushing through, their arms above them, carrying the coveted libations. The floor sparkled with confetti that rained down after someone purchased an insane amount of champagne. There were a few rappers huddled up in the corner. Young Money always had a table. I don't think Wayne was there, but definitely Mack Maine.

Scissors and Beard Bae were walking with me sandwiched directly between them, and I felt constant pressure that night to start the vibe. He was obviously attractive, and she's still the sexiest woman alive. When they could catch a glimpse, they looked each other up and down, sizing each other up. And it was super sexy because I knew them both well enough to know they liked what they saw.

Strangely, I surprised myself with how I was managing my jealousy. He's a taller, stronger, wealthier person than I am, let alone a MAN. She and I had to use hands, toys, fingers, and everything in between to experience penetration together, but he could give her the real thing. So why was this entire thing turning me on? My first encounter with this "sexy envy" continued throughout the night.

BB led us to a table one of his friends had arranged for him. At first, it was a little awkward—small talk about a bunch of nothing, light flirting, but nothing that would have led us to believe sex was to come a few hours later. In this scenario, I felt like the person bringing their friends together for the first time. I was the one starting the conversations. I was the one trying to foster mutual interest. But the vibe was still off, so I realized, *All right, I gotta break this shit up!*

I made some weak-ass excuse to go talk to a DJ or friend that I recognized; I just knew they needed a moment alone. Time to connect without me in the way. I was wasting time talking to whoever and watching them from across the club. He put his hand on the lower side of her back somewhat protectively, the way I knew he did when he liked someone. And Scissors was doing this sexy ass thing she does where she twirls her hair and smiles in her sexy-ass way. And I was like, *All right, she's pretty much DTF now, right? We can leave soon!*

After another hour of dancing, we decided to get some food before heading back to the hotel. When we were almost at the diner, the ultimate and best thing ever happened. Men rarely get to show how safe they can make women feel. That's what turns some of us on the most—feeling like they're our knight in shining armor. Scissors and I both love that shit. Nowadays, there are very few ways that a guy gets to show how much he can protect a woman, and honestly, this little asshole with stupid baggy pants walking by us on Collins Ave became the final catalyst for the threesome later.

He said something like, "DAAAAAMN, YOU GOT TWO HOES WITHCHA?" And when I tell you Beard Bae went straight into "WHO THE FUCK YOU TALKING TO?" mode—I could've filled a water bottle with how wet Scissors got after that.

Fast forward: the fries sucked, and we were ready to get the fuck up outta there. On the way to the hotel, he sat between us in the back of the car—a hand on each of our legs. Frankly, there was a whole energy shift. Now I, the orchestrator, was nervous! I couldn't remember the last time this bitch had got some dick, but she was ready to GO! On the other hand, I had experience in threesomes but never with someone I loved. What if this didn't go well? We were stuck with him for two more days! During the car ride, I realized that I had been so cocky and confident as the experienced one of the trio, but that just added to the pressure. It's the same anxiety I get whenever I sleep with someone new who knows I have a sex podcast. (Goddamn it, I have to find a way to get another tequila shot in me before this goes down.)

We got upstairs, and IDK if every lesbian relationship works this way, but Scissors and I always have these random homegirl bonding moments. We rushed to the bathroom to shower, and we checked in with each other while gushing about the night and our new knight.

"OMG! This is really gonna happen! Oh, I love you, baby. You look so pretty. BITCH! Hold up, fix my wig."

Finally, when we got to the bed, Beard Bae kissed her immediately. I can't remember if it was their first kiss, but I *can* remember not needing to be involved. I felt everything her body must have been feeling. Excitement, pleasure, nerves. It was a strange way of being intimately connected to Scissors. I remember her peeking her eyes open as her way of making sure that I was looking and that I was feeling comfortable. THIS NIGGA, on the other hand, was just happy to be there. LOL. He was consistently one of the tallest, sexiest, and most handsome men in any room. But that being said, this was still hers AND his first threesome!

In this moment, it could've gone one of two ways:

1. He could have expected us to serve him.
2. He could have been a giver.

AND THANK FUCKIN' GOD, I CHOSE A NUMBER TWO.

I sat on the edge of the bed and watched as they had a make out session. He was kissing her—one of those slow and sloppy kisses where you can watch a little bit of saliva as you pull apart from someone.

Again, I thought I'd feel jealous, hearing Scissors moan every time he squeezed her ass and her thighs. I believed my inner thoughts would be loud, like, *Are my hands not strong enough to grip her like that? Is she enjoying him more than me?* On the contrary, though, it made me wet. I felt this immense sense of pleasure in being able to watch her have an experience that I couldn't offer. I saw the way her eyes sparkled a little bit when she grabbed his dick through his boxers. The way she looked at me when she felt it and made sure to lock our gazes while he was growing harder in her hands.

Finally, after being a fly on the wall and enjoying myself, I realized my lack of participation could have come off as jealousy. So I started to kiss them.

My ultimate fantasy had always been getting fucked while giving head. In all honesty, I didn't give a damn if it was a man or woman on either end, but it would have fulfilled the giving and pleasing side of me. Scissors was lying down, and we both started to go down on her. I remember her pussy being his and my first kiss back in the hotel room. Bae and I just devoured her, and it was the sexiest fucking thing I could have imagined. I remember my eyes being closed and my mouth filling up with her flavor. I could taste more of her than usual—her pussy was creaming, and the smell of her pheromones made her irresistible to me and Beard Bae.

She kept moaning so loudly that I was almost overstimulated with how horny I was, the constant sound of her, my body throbbing. Then Beard Bae stopped and got behind me; he was so fucking hard that it felt like his dick was bigger than it had ever been before. At this point in my life, gazing someone in the eye was a difficult thing for me to do, but I remember looking up at Scissors in the most submissive way. She stroked my face. It was this weird start to my role in this scenario, from the voyeur to being their bottom. But even though my fantasy was coming true, I found that I wanted to trade places with Scissors. I wanted to watch her.

He stopped, and we went down on him together before he started fucking Scissors. She was on her back with her legs spread in the air as he slid into her, missionary. I remember being able to smell his musk. Not in this smelly, I-just-got-done-playing-basketball type of way, but a real animalistic pheromone that just comes out of a man when he's super fucking horny. I was so desperate to watch that I silently prayed that they would forget I was there and enjoy each other.

She kept pulling me by my waist to sit on her face, but I really just wanted to concentrate on this moment of watching them. I got on top of her and kind of hovered over her stomach so that she could taste me. I hated that for the few moments when she went down on me, her moaning got muffled. I wanted her to immerse herself in this experience and enjoy him fully. I needed to sit in that experience I kept having. I had this gut feeling of jealousy and arousal mixed with happiness. It was like I was cuckolding and participating at the same time. My negative emotions associated with jealousy became clear right then and there. Jealousy *can* trigger excitement; jealousy *is* temporary, and *my* jealousy was *my* source of pleasure.

That was when I thought my post-nut clarity should have kicked in. How could I have sat there and let my girlfriend fuck my FWB and just become a literal pawn in their pretty much TWOSOME!

I was literally their cum cleanup.

And I loved every fucking second of it.

All the countless love songs about heartbreak were debunked for me after this experience. This night set the tone for the standard of my relationships today. I can't go back to the vanilla way of life. "Just the two of us." Eh . . . more like just the two of us + her on the weekends?

The weird thing is that my childhood ideals of what my relationships would look like did not necessarily change. There are just more people in the picture than I'd originally imagined, and that feels aligned with who I currently am. I am now in a relationship where I am committed to a male partner, but we are an ethically non-monogamous couple.

Ethical non-monogamy is a term for relationships where all partners openly consent to romantic, intimate, and/or sexual relationships with multiple people.

Happiness is attainable with other partners involved. I know this because this is my lived experience. I've seen them intertwined and tangled up in my bed together. I've tasted them both and enjoyed their different flavors. I've touched them, the different textures, the smooth and the rough, and I've felt joy at the endless options. Our sexual desires are not synonymous with loyalty to the person we choose to commit our lives to.

For this kind of relationship to work, honesty is the rule. If you are going to be non-monogamous, open communication is the key. If you have been cheated on, the person lying to you may not feel safe enough to express their urges to you, because we have been conditioned to believe that our partner having eyes for someone else means that we are no longer loved. Now, I am not siding with liars; as you will learn in other chapters, I've also been victim to many disappointments from being lied to. But it's a bit of a vicious cycle.

Although the act is selfish, I believe some liars think their lies protect their partners from hurt feelings. According to *Psychology Today*, infidelity can actually be a form of self-exploration. "They're not looking for another person; they're looking for hidden versions of themselves," says Robert Weiss, who is the author of several books that help support male sex addicts and their families in healing.[3] Those "liars" are selfish for being with someone that simply isn't interested in the lifestyle that they want. But how can someone know that if they don't give their partner the chance to know who they are?

This doesn't mean you should LET your person cheat on you, but you should keep an open dialogue about where you both are really at. In her groundbreaking book *Mating in Captivity*, Esther Perel said it best: "We ground ourselves in familiarity, and perhaps achieve a peaceful domestic arrangement, but in the process we orchestrate boredom. The verve of the relationship collapses under the weight of all that control. Stultified, couples are left wondering, 'What ever happened to fun? What ever happened to excitement, to transcendence, to awe?'"[4]

I hope there is a day when no one thinks commitment is the end of our fun. My current partner recently told me that if we ever get married, he will skip out on a bachelor party because it implies he'd act differently after being married. My man doesn't need a night away with his boys to let loose because he has a partner with whom he can be himself. And I feel the same way.

I now know that being the only sexual partner means nothing about someone's love for me. I'm not going to be left alone just because I decide to have a sexual experience with someone outside of our duo. Sex isn't the determining factor in commitment for me anymore. I have genuinely become someone who enjoys another person's happiness and pleasures. I haven't accepted being cheated on, but I have invited what's usually a solo experience into my own bedroom.

I'm also willing to share my current relationship nonnegotiables within our ethically non-monogamous dynamic.

CONDOMS. ALWAYS—Any breach of this is a blatant disrespect to our health and free will. This is 100 percent nonnegotiable.
NO SLEEPOVERS—My personal favorite way to connect is our alone time sleeping together, so we chose to keep this sacred.

OVERRIDE—At any point when a third party makes either of us uncomfortable, insecure, or unsafe, the relationship with the third party will be ended, no questions asked.

And over the years we may add more rules. For now, I have found that these three components are simple yet strict enough to keep my heart in a safe situation with the partners I have chosen to be with. For me, the central relationship should always be a priority, with sexual desires for others being secondary to that.

Be open to the idea that there IS someone for everyone. Maybe more than one someone sometimes. ;-) I'm not saying that when you finish this chapter, you should start a threesome group chat, but maybe . . . yOU SHoUld!

Patriarchal Bullshit

"The great question that has never been answered
and which I have not yet been able to answer,
despite my thirty years of research into the
feminine soul, is 'What does a woman want?'"
—Sigmund Freud (to Marie Bonaparte)[1]

Matriarchal Reply

"We have been raised to fear the yes within ourselves, our
deepest cravings. But, once recognized, those which do not
enhance our future lose their power and can be altered. The
fear of our desires keeps them suspect and indiscriminately
powerful, for to suppress any truth is to give it strength
beyond endurance. The fear that we cannot grow beyond
whatever distortions we may find within ourselves keeps us
docile and loyal and obedient, externally defined, and leads
us to accept many facets of our oppression as women."
—Audre Lorde
(author of *Sister Outsider: Essays and Speeches*)[2]

DID YOU KNOW YOU CAN FIND UNICORNS IN MEXICO?

« MANDII B »

DESPITE TRYING HARD to ignore other people's opinions, we are heavily influenced and affected by how society and our peers view us. It often affects how we dress, talk, and express or suppress emotions. Even more, the unsolicited opinions of our direct circle and society have an impact on who we may choose to date, the decisions we make in relationships, and how we express our sexuality. Frequently, we find ourselves either hiding or exaggerating the truth about our dating and sex lives for fear of being judged, labeled, or shamed by our family, friends, and the world. Even in grade school, nobody wants to be known as the girl who is "easy," "fast," or the "hoe of the school." Exploring yourself alone and with partners becomes a game of hide-and-seek—hiding from those who would deem your behavior promiscuous while also seeking to find yourself through sexual exploration, love, and heartbreak.

Think about how many times you would have left the club with the hot guy who flirted with you all night, if you didn't worry your friends would judge you for having a one-night stand. Was there a time when you dated someone and knew your parents would hate them, so you sabotaged the relationship on purpose? I don't believe we realize how often we allow others to place us in the prisons we find ourselves trying to escape from well into our adulthood. I use the word "allow" because many of us, without knowing it at all, possess the key to escape these prisons. We must overcome the fear of what others may think of us if we want to unabashedly live the life we want for ourselves.

Now, before I help you find ways to get yourself out of the damn Prison of Other People's Opinions, I'm going to take you on a trip with me.

I was floating in the center of a crystalline ocean; I couldn't believe I'd booked a trip to Mexico alone. I was depleted from the emotional roller coaster I couldn't get off with my boyfriend at the time. I'd have done anything to stop the heavy throbbing pain that had replaced the beating of my heart and the waves of nausea that had replaced the feeling of butterflies. Amidst this breakup, I was also experiencing seasonal burnout. The podcast was doing great, but Weezy and I could have been in a better place. I was heavily involved in other projects that seemed debilitating. My work and personal life were unbalanced, and I just needed a quick escape. I needed a break.

I'd decided that taking a solo vacation to Cancún was what I needed to get over all the bullshit that life was throwing in my face at once. I thought, *FUCK IT! I'm going to go on a trip by myself and for myself. I'm going to read books, relax, go to sleep, lay by the pool, drink fucking mojitos all day long, and then REPEAT.* This was going to be my trip of self-revival, where I would start the healing process and regroup. The books I'd brought on my trip were *The Four Agreements: A Practical Guide to Personal Freedom*, a self-help book by Don Miguel Ruiz, and *Set Boundaries, Find Peace* by Nedra Glover Tawwab. I had also brought a blank journal in which I anticipated beginning my writing journey of healing. I was ready to learn to set healthy boundaries, find inner peace, and break the damn cycle of whatever trauma was affecting me within my interpersonal relationships. This would be my Black girl version of *Eat Pray Love.*

I checked in breezily, intending to enter Zen mode immediately. But almost as soon as I'd arrived at my high-end, all-inclusive hotel, I realized I had chosen the wrong place. This hotel spawned a party that appeared to blend *BET's Spring Bling* with one of those *Girls Gone Wild* DVDs. Since I was annoyed at my choice of hotel, I decided to get out of there and check something off my bucket list that I'd always wanted to do. I had wanted to swim with whale sharks on a trip to South Africa, and my friends had looked at me like I was batshit crazy. I had convinced them to ride a truck with no windows on the safari, where we encountered lions and tigers and bears (OH MY!), but they had no interest in helping me knock sharks off my list of things I just had to do. Since this was my solo-cation, I decided to book the one-hundred-forty-dollar whale shark excursion and make my escape simultaneously.

The following day, I had a super early breakfast and went to the pier because I had to be there by 8 a.m. I was fairly confident about taking another dive into the ocean's deep waters. I had been snorkeling in the waters of Thailand and swum with the fish in the Caribbean. How different could this be? I felt I was prepared to do the damn thang.

We were told that we had half an hour until we got to the spot where we'd do our dive. I looked around the boat and felt alone. No one looked like anyone I'd want to talk to; even if they had, I was the only person who didn't speak Spanish. I headed to an empty seat in the back of the boat and, in true vacation fashion, asked for a cerveza. I may not know much Spanish, but I'll be damned if I don't know how to ask for a beer. I decided to stay alone on the back of the boat; I looked out and saw colorful fish and dolphins leaping over the waves. I stuck my hand out, feeling the water splash, thinking, *Bitch, you literally just took yourself on a fucking vacation.* I reminded myself that with all the hard work came rewards.

We finally reached the whale sharks' habitat, and I put on my wetsuit, flippers, and snorkel. I looked over the side of the boat nervously because I could see these whale sharks coming up out of the water with their gigantic mouths wide open. I thought, *Now, bitchhh, what the hell were you thinkin'?*

It was my turn and I dove in, and the guide motioned for me to go under. I couldn't believe that I was swimming with the fucking whale sharks! They were big and gray and had white speckles. I looked to my right and decided to come back up because the whale shark right next to me was giant as fuck. Yup! I was a whole chicken shit! That thang scared me as it briskly swam next to me, the size of two school buses combined. We were supposed to do three jumps, but after one, I was finished. I could say I had done it. I had my video as evidence. That was enough for me. I decided to go back to the boat and have another beer. By this time, tons of people were jumping in the water to swim with what appeared to be over a dozen whale sharks, while I relaxed with my cerveza.

It was finally time for everyone to return to our boat. The next stop was an idyllic island called Isla Mujeres. As the ship started to pull toward the island, I saw the sandy white beach, and the water sparkled every shade of blue. It was breathtaking. Tons of families were laid out across their towels with umbrellas. Tiki huts and restaurants lined the coastline, and I fell in love with the place—before I fell in love with the sight of something else. As we got closer to dropping the anchor, I spotted something on the beach that was even more captivating: a huge, tall, dark-skinned man with blue shorts and no shirt walking with this short, thick-ass girl who wore a red one-piece swimsuit. She had the body that I would've loved to see represented on *Baywatch,* and she damn sure did that swimsuit justice. Looking at them, I couldn't help but think how much they resembled me and my ex. And for a second, I let myself get all in my feelings; I was like, *Damn, that's what we look like. I wish I was here with him.* And reallllll damn quick, I had to snap myself out of that shit! I wouldn't allow him to ruin what I had set out to do for me.

The boat docked, and I went straight toward the tiki bar a little way down the beach. Our excursion didn't have any liquor, so even though we were supposed to stay close to the boat because we were only there for thirty or forty minutes, I was ready to get myself a real drink. I walked inside the hut, and who was standing there ordering their drinks? As it turned out, this couple was even better-looking up close. They finished ordering, and the bartender was taking forever, so we just stood there and waited around. That was when I decided to tell the woman how beautiful she was. She had an olive complexion; long, dirty-blond loose curls damp from the ocean; and big dark-brown eyes I could drown in. She smiled and thanked me before complimenting me back. Their drinks arrived, and the couple returned to the beach to enjoy the water and sun. It was finally my turn to order, and my wheels were spinning, so I thought, *YOLO!* I ordered three shots, then headed down the sand toward them. This was my moment to shoot my shot.

I want to pause my story here. Because some of you may think a man is supposed to make the first move. As a woman, how do you "shoot your shot"? Listen, a big part of overcoming the fear of dating, sex, and relationships is letting all of THE BULLSHIT RULES go and accepting the possibility of rejection. We all fear rejection because it reflects the other person's opinion of us.

When "shooting your shot," these are the things I remember so I can be brave.

THE WORST THING THEY CAN SAY IS NO—You enjoy the power of saying no to others, so allow others that same autonomy and be okay with receiving it.

EVERYONE IS NOT FOR EVERYONE—Every person you find attractive is NOT a potential partner. Rejection is normal! If a person is uninterested in you, don't take it personally. Plenty more fish are in the sea, and it's possible that person can be in your life in some other capacity.

IT IS FINE TO BE CORNY (SOMETIMES)—Start the conversation with a joke or a bad pickup line that can break the ice. You can both laugh about how bad the joke was, and then you can lean in next with a compliment. If that's too straightforward for you, reference a drink on the menu or the sports game on the television screen.

EMBARRASSMENT TYPICALLY DOESN'T LAST VERY LONG—Have you ever jumped into a cold plunge or off a boat into the ocean and felt the shock hit your body, only for the water to feel perfect soon after? Be fine with laughing at yourself and know that embarrassment is a feeling we don't have to sit with for long. It's not the end of the world. Managing your embarrassment can help you grow. Get a grip on it and it will assist in your confidence to go after what and WHO you want.

The couple were pretty surprised when I approached them, said hello, and offered them both tequila. We did the shots and started talking, and I found out they were married and were in Mexico to celebrate the husband's thirty-fifth birthday. I couldn't help but stare at him because he was my exact type. I was extremely attracted to them both.

The sun was beating down and getting extremely hot on our melanated skin, so we all got into the water to cool off. It turned out they also lived in New York; we talked about life in the city and how they'd met. The conversation was easy and natural, and I enjoyed spending time with them. He said he'd be right back and got out of the water. She and I continued to talk, and even though he was gone, speaking alone with her felt natural. It was almost like I already knew them.

The man reappeared with three more shots. "Well, if you are going to buy us a shot, we must return the favor," he said with a smile of mischief.

I peered over to my tour boat and realized the crew was all heading back to it. It was time to leave.

"Damn, I'm only here for a little bit because I'm staying in Cancún. My boat is about to leave, so I'd better head back."

They both looked disappointed. I hated that our time had to be cut short. They shared the same sentiment. I realized that I wanted to stay. I had never been to this island and wanted the opportunity to explore. Now, yes, I also wanted to explore both their bodies, but I didn't think it'd actually go that far! I genuinely wanted to see what this small island of beauty offered. I had never left a tour midway through, but I made up my mind without anyone's opinions or needs but my own to be met. I trekked back to the boat, got my belongings, negotiated a rate for my overpriced pictures and videos with the whale sharks, and told them I wouldn't be completing the tour and would find my own way back to the mainland. Then I quickly rejoined my new "friends."

They'd planned to go beach club hopping, and now I was the third wheel along for the ride. We hit up two or three beach clubs. I remember all of us getting a little hungry, so we ate lunch at one of the outdoor seated areas. I was struck by how he treated his wife with reverence and kindness. He seemed to want to make sure that she was always good, and eventually, he started to treat me the same way. He made sure to lead by holding a great deal of consideration for what the two of us wanted. He took care of us and paid for everything, which was crazy because this was his birthday trip. We were having an incredible time together, bouncing from place to place, day drinking, laughing, and talking, and eventually, the conversation evolved. We finally started to talk about sex.

Talking to people about sex and making them feel comfortable is obviously one of my strong suits, so I asked the wife if she'd ever been with a woman. She smiled and told me she was no rookie in the lady pond. We talked about what we'd done and hadn't done. She shared that she had been in a threesome with two other women that she'd thoroughly enjoyed. We started talking about our fantasies and what we wanted to try.

To many people, talking about sex too soon or oversharing on a date is another way in which we show up with our fear of what someone else may think of us. Over the years, I've found it to be the quickest indicator of someone who may not be my type. Now, while I do have a sex podcast, I, too, don't necessarily find it comfortable to have these conversations in every setting or with just anybody.

Here are some questions to ask yourself before having a conversation regarding your sexual desires or history:

DO I WANT TO FUCK THIS PERSON?—This should be the FIRST question you ask yourself. As women, I think we know fairly early if we're going to give it up. If you do not feel that you'd ever fuck this individual, feel free to say you are uncomfortable with the conversation. You can always revisit this later. If you do want to fuck this person, repeat after me: "My desires and pleasure matter more to me than this person's thoughts about me."

DO I FIND THIS PERSON TO BE SEXUALLY COMPATIBLE WITH MY NEEDS AND DESIRES?—If you find yourself in conversation with someone who doesn't seem to be sexually compatible by their responses or previous experiences, be okay with knowing that this may be a big waste of time if you do make it to the bedroom. Stand firm in what you like and be very aware of how they respond to your inquiries.

HOW DO I FEEL THE MOST COMFORTABLE DISCUSSING SEX?—You may have difficulty expressing your sexual needs and fantasies to someone you don't know well. Perhaps you feel more comfortable writing them down and conversing over text messages. Ease into the conversation by showing examples of the things you are into. You can do this by referencing porn clips or articles. Don't feel pressured to have this conversation in a setting that prevents you from being clear or understood.

The three of us had a conversation where everything flowed, and I trusted my gut. I knew we would all be sexually compatible. They already had dinner reservations for that night and needed to return to their hotel. I figured I should find my way to the ferry and get back to my hotel, but they explained that I still had plenty of time to catch the last ferry and could join them for dinner. As you can imagine by now, the sexual tension was off the charts, and so I gladly obliged. We got back to their place, and the husband went to the balcony to fill up the room's jacuzzi. I suggested we shower first to rinse off the sand from a full day on the beach.

And this is where things really started to kick off. I got into the shower and told The Wife she should come in with me. I started washing her hair and soaping up her body. To this day, that alone was one of the most sensual experiences I've had. Then, she and I asked The Husband to join us. He was hesitant and seemed to not believe our request. He finally decided to get in and joined me in washing the sand off his partner's body. We then switched to washing him, watching the soapy suds drip off his body and swirl into the drain below us.

Then, in unison, we began taking turns fitting him into our mouths. We went back and forth from his magnificent, throbbing dick to each other's mouths to be sure we both tasted him in every which way. As she continued pleasing her partner, I couldn't wait to begin tasting her. While she devoured his now strong and long member, I lowered myself onto the cold tiled floor and lifted her hips to place her directly on my face. The shower was still going, so I was tasting her while also trying not to drown from the water cascading down her body to where my nose and mouth rested in between her thighs.

We left the bathroom and took our soaking-wet bodies to the

bedroom. We attempted to dry off as much as possible, but my body was still somewhat damp as we quickly plummeted onto the bed to continue. He and I both started to please her together. We took turns going in what felt like an assembly line down her soft, curvy body. It began with a deep, passionate kiss where our tongues danced with one another. Those kisses left her mouth and began the trail down to her neck before making a pit stop on her breast. Her breasts were full, and her areolas were light brown against the sun-kissed tan she had gotten from being on the beach all day.

I remember looking in her eyes as I traveled down to her sweet spot. I grabbed her hips to lift her leaking pussy up in an effort to reach every crevice possible. She tasted sweet. I ate her like she was my last meal on death row. My tongue was working like it had trained for a marathon. I didn't want to stop.

Then, they both started devouring me. I usually get pleasure out of giving it. I enjoy pleasing someone and hearing their moans as I do what I know I do very well. But I allowed myself to sink into the now damp white sheets on the bed to take in being a Pillow Princess, if only for a few minutes. We passionately kissed while he went back and forth between putting each of my breasts into his mouth. He reached down to feel how wet I had become. I was a leaking fucking faucet, you hear me? I remember seeing them lock eyes. It was like she read his mind. He wanted to feel me from the inside and proceeded cautiously. She nodded to grant all the permission he had been seeking.

Over the next thirty minutes, we both shared his long, girthy dick. At one point, I slid my body under hers as she was taking him from the back. This was my chance to taste them both in unison while giving her the pleasure of licking her clit as he slid in and out of her. He was patient, catching his breath to ensure we both came before he did. It was an even exchange of consideration between us all. We wanted each of us to be in ecstasy and to reach orgasm before ending the show. Mission accomplished.

Once he finally came, he was so winded. It was hot, and even though the A/C was on, we'd steamed up the room's sliding glass door with our deep, warm breaths. It seemed like he wanted a moment to wake himself up from the dream he was sure he was in. *Is this real fuckin' life?* He stood up and went into the bathroom. She and I were lying in the big bed, cuddled up together. We heard the water run. He came back with warm rags for each of us. He tossed them onto the bed before stroking his dick into the warm towel he'd prepared for himself. His body was so fuckin' chiseled as he stood towering over the both of us with his 6'5" frame. He smiled, then couldn't help himself. Continuing to look puzzled, he blurted out, "Did y'all plan this? You all know each other, don't you?"

He was so blown away by the experience that he thought it couldn't have happened by chance. He continued with his line of questioning. "Where did you two meet?" He became convinced that the wife must have planned this as part of his birthday present. He thought it had been a setup because it was just too fucking perfect and magical. Things like this did not usually just happen in real life, even to me, and I have experienced some pretty incredible shit. On a trip where I had convinced myself that I needed complete solace, here I was, laid up with not one, but two people who made me feel safe and at peace.

In hindsight, I do recognize how lucky I was to be a part of such a beautiful and unexpected sexual experience without having "the talk." We hadn't discussed our boundaries, kinks, traumas, or sexual desires with one another. There were very few words exchanged before the swapping of bodily fluids. These talks are typically foundational to setting yourself up for success when adding a third or becoming a third in the bedroom. I have been fortunate to engage in group sex, which often ends in bliss. However, I would be doing you a disservice if I didn't share what typically leads to these experiences being so positive. Before having group sex, you should be considerate of all parties involved and have the following conversations:

BOUNDARIES FOR THE COUPLE—If you want to bring in a third party, a conversation MUST be had with your partner around your boundaries. Discuss what acts are off-limits and what could ruin the vibe. You must be honest with yourself. Do you consider your partner kissing someone to be too intimate? What measures of protection do you plan to use? Will you require recent test results? Being on the same page with your partner is essential.

BOUNDARIES FOR THE THIRD—Suppose you are the third person joining an established duo. In that case, it is vital to know the boundaries they have established and check in before and during with both parties with more attention going to the person of the same sex. Jealousy often arises, and it's crucial to reassure the same-sex person in a FFM threesome that you are not in competition and are pleased to be a part of this experience with both individuals.

KINKS—It is essential to ask a person their kinks and the things that they enjoy during sex, and to share your own in return. Whether you like to be slapped, spit on, or even pissed on, it should be clear what things turn you both on and off before bringing it to the bed. Thinking of every scenario can be challenging, so I suggest creating a safeword. A safeword is a word that anyone can use during play that completely stops whatever is happening. It's wise to steer clear of words like "stop," "no," or "slower," and to use a word that would not often come up naturally. A word like "pineapples" is a good example, but you can pick any word you all agree to.

TRAUMAS—Traumas can be a difficult conversation topic out the gate with people. However, the last thing anyone wants during a sexual experience is to trigger someone or to be triggered by a past trauma. Perhaps the person you are about to engage with has a trauma around being choked or hearing a specific word. No need to go into deep detail; however, if you know what your trigger is, be sure that you share that with the people you are about to be intimate with.

I want to reiterate that this was different from how my younger self sought validation. This experience was not about being affirmed by other people at all. This experience was about releasing my fear of rejection and society's expectations of me, living in the moment, and doing exactly whatever the fuck it was I wanted to do.

It was getting late, and we realized they would miss their dinner reservation if they didn't get ready. I was, once again, about to go and find my way to the ferry when they said no, come to dinner with us instead. I wasn't prepared to go anywhere that wasn't casual since I'd shown up on the island in my bathing suit and shorts. I told them, "I don't have anything to wear." The wife was not hesitant to note that we were similar in size before she pulled out a flowy black blouse and a pair of striped shorts for me.

That evening at the table, I thought, *Wow. I'm really on a date with two people right now.* I was interested in both of them, and both of them were interested in me. It felt so good and so natural that my brain was like, *What the fuck is this?* It was so interesting that I found this feeling of safety and complete ease with two strangers. And then I decided to say "fuck it" yet again. I let myself just be. It was freeing and liberating. I realized how much I wished we would all allow ourselves to "be" more. I removed the fears of what society may think of this random vacation rendezvous. I disregarded any judgment that may have come from any of my friends. I chose to live in bliss on this tranquil, beautiful island with this gorgeous couple and take in the moment for what it was. It was me living.

After dinner, we wanted to go clubbing, but we were all too fucking exhausted. So we went back to their hotel and climbed back into the big California king bed together. We lay there that night cuddling and watching *The Office*. Oh yeah, and WE DID HAVE SEX AGAIN, OF COURSE! I fell asleep between them, big spooning The Wife while being held by The Husband. It was the perfect mix of sex and intimacy.

The next morning, we had breakfast, and they asked if I'd like to spend the day touring the island with them. On Isla Mujeres, you can rent golf carts and drive around to restaurants and shops. During the ride, I watched as each house became grander and more enormous and saw the small convenience stores where the locals purchased their groceries. There was a boutique hotel the couple wanted to check out, and it was breathtaking. I felt like I was in Fiji, with water so clear that I could see straight to the bottom. The place had these giant pools with cascading waterfalls and little alcoves in which you could relax. We stayed there for most of the day, smoking hookah, eating until we couldn't eat anymore, and jumping between the ocean's saltiness and the swimming pool's coolness. It felt like we had disappeared into an even more enchanted island getaway. Then we finally left to catch the sunset together. This was the most romantic day I'd had in an extremely long time. At that moment, I wanted to be with them both forever.

Besides the memories I had made on this tiny island over the past thirty hours, I didn't have much to leave with. I only ever spoke to the couple two more times, one time to ask their permission to talk about them on the podcast and when they let me know they listened. They told me they'd enjoyed the episode. They thanked me for ensuring they remained anonymous but also shared the sentiments of how magical our weekend together felt to them. We talked about them taking me to their favorite seafood place in New Jersey, but it has yet to happen. Reality set back in. We were back home to our everyday lives, and briefly after this trip I hopped back onto the emotional roller-coaster ride of my on-again-off-again relationship.

This story has become a fantasy to me—one where I got everything I could've wanted and asked for. I'd integrated perfectly into this couple without any way of knowing that I could. None of us are given the manual on how to bag a couple and become a unicorn. And maybe that's part of why I never saw them again. The idea of embracing and making love to two people with respect and intimacy seems like a fallacy. Others often shun the idea of allowing your partner access to someone else. Intimacy and affection are customarily taken off the menu as these acts of love typically bring out a partner's insecurities. I needed to remember that this feeling could exist, even if it was only possible for two days. I got into my head about this truly being something that could exist in a long-term setting. Would their friends and family even accept them having a whole girlfriend? Did they only feel comfortable inviting me in because they were on a trip with no other eyes?

I got to experience something that so many people never get to: getting out of their heads and going after what they want. I did something that I would have never done on a trip with other people. I said, "Fuck feeling embarrassed," and did that shit! I realized the importance of trying new things and being open but also truthful to myself. I learned the true meaning of the motto "You only live once." I'm not saying that it will always work out perfectly, but you only know once you give yourself the chance to try.

Patriarchal Bullshit
"Feminism [. . .] encourages women to leave
their husbands, kill their children, practice witchcraft,
destroy capitalism, and become lesbians."
—Pat Robertson (reverend and religious broadcaster)[1]

Matriarchal Reply
"I have the freedom to like who I like.
If I like a guy, that doesn't mean I'm straight.
If I like a girl, that doesn't mean I'm a lesbian.
Just let me be and let me love who I want
to without trying to categorize me."
—Demi Burnett (American television personality,
season 23 of *The Bachelor*)[2]

ARE SCISSORS ONLY FOR ARTS AND CRAFTS?

« WEEZYWTF »

MY MOM MENTIONED to me once that she knew I was kinda gay from how I treated my female friends when I was a kid. I was very clingy and private when I was around them. I wanted to stay hidden with them behind locked doors, and I was overly sad whenever they left our house. "Kinda gay" is my favorite way to describe my sexuality—no disrespect to the LGBTQIA+s, but I'm KG (kinda gay).

My preferred way of gayness when I was ten was grinding on the neighbor's daughter. We would wear panties and rub on each other while a sex scene in a movie we rented at Blockbuster played. Sometimes I didn't even need the sex. Just a flash of breasts was good enough for me, like Nadia's from *American Pie* or even the quick titties in *Coming to America*. Thankfully, it takes a lot more to get me off now. Or, wait, maybe not . . .

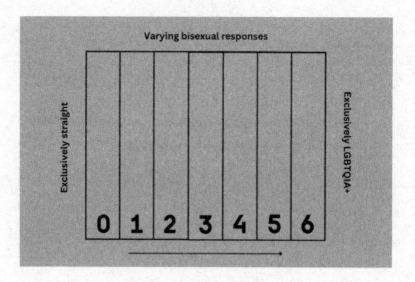

I learned about the Kinsey Scale, also known as the Heterosexual–Homosexual Rating Scale, in the early days of the podcast. It is a tool developed by Dr. Alfred Kinsey and his colleagues in the mid-twentieth century to describe a person's sexual orientation. The scale ranges from 0 to 6, with an additional category of "X" for those who are asexual.[3]

Here's our version of the scale:

> 0: Exclusively straight with no LGBTQIA+ experiences or feelings.
>
> 1: Predominantly straight, only incidentally LGBTQIA+.
>
> 2: Predominantly straight, but more than incidentally LGBTQIA+.
>
> 3: Equally straight and LGBTQIA+.
>
> 4: Predominantly LGBTQIA+, but more than incidentally straight.

5: Predominantly LGBTQIA+, only incidentally straight.

6: Exclusively LGBTQIA+ with no straight experiences or feelings.

And then there is X: which is not traditionally shared on the scale.

X: No socio-sexual contacts or reactions (asexual).

Apparently, none of us are super straight or super gay. For me, my gayness depended on how hot you were! At home, my porn searches got increasingly more raunchy as my exploration went on, and girl-on-girl videos were always at the top of the list during my teenage years. Strap-on, pussy licking, fingering, tribbing, scissoring, and sometimes even breastfeeding. I just wanted to see women in every single scenario. What I learned after living kinda gay for a few years was that lesbian porn was made for the male gaze. All the beauty, the crazy moaning, the back arching—that shit wasn't fuckin' real.

The first pussy I ever tasted was this gorgeous Dominican woman's; she was everything I would have described a video vixen to look like. She had the perfect body, long dark hair, and a smile that made everyone weak. She was only four years older than me but so overtly sexual that I think she pulled the gay out of me. Maybe she knew I was always crushing on her, or perhaps she was just super horny. She would find a way to get naked in front of me, even if we weren't changing clothes. She'd talk about how hot it was outside and take off her top, rub her breasts, and giggle at how uncomfortable it made me. I think part of her attraction to me was how nervous I was around her. I've found that when I am really into someone, I get super-duper shy around them.

She had the body the Instagram BBL girls dream of; her ass-to-waist ratio was so insane you almost felt like it wasn't real. She smelled like candy and always wore this pink-tinted lip gloss to match that aesthetic. When we went out together, I would watch men damn near fall over. I always believed it was because she was the embodiment of perfection. She wasn't just beautiful; she had the personality to match. Guys would gawk at her crazy fat ass and say something crude, and she would smile and say something like, "Is that how your mother taught you to speak to ladies? I hope you treat the next woman better!" winking as she walked away.

I loved everything about her attitude. Sometimes she held on to my waist in clubs to show she was spoken for. I could only think, *Who's really gonna believe she's with me???* She would dance with me slowly, not caring who watched, and if the liquor and molly were flowing strong enough, she'd kiss me. I became obsessed with her kisses. She would always grab my face when she was ready for one, right under the chin, and pucker her lips like a mother and child would kiss goodbye. Then, after she warmed me up with pecks, it was full-on tongue and make outs. I understand how juvenile this sentiment may sound to you, considering you picked up a book about sex. But that's what her kisses were like. They were good enough for me to masturbate to when I'd drive myself home after the clubs. I wouldn't even want to shower after leaving her so that I could still smell the candy and play with the red lipstick all over my face. If you ask me, my nineteen-year-old self could have handled just the kissing and been happy. I used to be scared of what actual sex may be like. How would I even be good at it?

The two of us drove up to Tampa one night to hit up the club

Blue Martini. It was twenty-one and up, but luckily, she had an older sister with an ID I could use to get in. We got EXTRA drunk that night—amaretto sours, lemon drops, or whatever was free. She was very handsy with me for the first time with no words spoken. She'd flick one of my nipples and giggle or find ways to put her hands up my dress and touch the edge of my thong. I was so nervous about that night finally being the night, so I spent an extra long time during every bathroom trip to make sure my pussy was wiped clean and ready for whatever was to come.

When we left the club, she kissed me in the parking lot in a way that let me know our friendship was about to change. She told me we were going to a friend's house and not to be nervous. When we arrived, a real brolic dark-skinned man opened up the door and said, "Well damn all right, den!" in the most country-ass accent possible. He was a football player she was sleeping with between her on-and-off-again boyfriend. He was cute, but I was frankly so invested in her at the time that I would have done whatever she told me. We went into his bedroom while his friends played video games in the living room. Since we were already waiting, he rushed his homeboys to leave.

Was this about to be my first threesome AND my first time eating pussy??? Nah, this was too fucking much to handle in one night. I started to get a little nervous, saying how drunk I was, hoping she'd let me bail out. But instead, she told me to relax as she started to undress and take her panties off. I mirrored exactly what she was doing since, after all, she was the older woman in this scenario.

She got onto the bed, parted her legs, and put her fingers up inside her pussy. She made room for me to come next to her, and since I was too intimidated to touch her, I just started to touch myself, too. We kissed for a longggggg time, letting our tongues just rest in each other's mouths while we moaned and fucked ourselves. The closer I got to making myself cum, the braver I became. I got in between her legs, staring at her, smelling her, scared of what the taste would be like and worried I wouldn't know what to do when I was down there. She was waxed and super smooth. I used two fingers in the shape of a peace sign to spread her lips apart, and to my surprise, she was pierced!

Now, my dear reader, I'm not sure if you have ever seen a pierced vagina, but as rare as they are, imagine it being the first one you ever put in your mouth! I was overwhelmed, but I could tackle most challenges, so I was not about to let that little hoop ring defeat me. I started to play with her clit with my hand first, and I listened to her voice begin to get breathy the harder I touched her. Breath is always a telltale sign of whether you're doing a good job, and I love being a good listener. I let her body be my teacher. I remembered a '90s movie said to spell the alphabet out with your tongue, and I literally did that.

I spelled *A*, *B*, *C*, *D*, and *E*, making sure not to say it out loud. She loved it; she kept grabbing my hair, squeezing her legs over my face, and burying me deeper inside her pussy. I loved how messy I was getting from her wetness and my own spit. It was so satisfying to me that I even started to touch myself while I ate her pussy. I was so close to making myself orgasm when I heard her gasp and release her grip on me as the door opened. He was right behind me, watching.

My first time with a woman was amazing. Even if a man did come in between us to take all the shine, pussy became something I always had a craving for. I spent my fair share of weekends making out with or fucking random girls I met. My boyfriend now tells me all the time that I have masculine energy, and although I hate hearing that, I believe it to be the reason girls flock to me. I find myself constantly being a girl's "first," which I really don't care for. Straight girls discover that I'm an easy way in. Once I got a girlfriend, though, the attention from women got even worse.

I can't remember exactly "how" I met Scissors in high school, but I knew she would be a special person in my life. It wasn't just the sex with her, even though that's what all my homeboys wanted to think about. She was beautiful and had sort of an elitist and bratty attitude that I was oddly attracted to. When we became friends, we almost immediately started a sexual relationship. It wasn't necessarily our entire dynamic, but it was one that she initiated while I longed for more. We were both sleeping with a guy outside of each other, but everyone around town had figured out that we were secretly fucking. I hated that I was a secret to her. She was the first person I ever snuck out of bed to put on makeup for in the morning. She was one of those girly girls, and I would have done anything to be like her. Not because I wanted to look like her, but because I wanted her to see herself in me.

The day I fell in love with her coincided with a family tragedy. It was my grandma's seventy-fifth birthday party, and my mom threw a casino night at our house for her. I'd told my mother I was bringing Scissors over the night before, and she'd said, "Oh God, honey, not tonight; we can tell everyone you're gay tomorrow. Just let her get introduced. Start slow. I have so much running around and so much food to make I can't handle this right now!"

I held Scissors's hand as we walked in the door and introduced her to my parents and all their hoity-toity friends; I remember my dad's face and everyone's weirdness about how attached we were. I felt so proud to have this half-step out of the closet around people so close to me. My mom has forever been a supporter and just all around someone who doesn't care about sexual orientation, but it was vital for me to take that more significant leap in front of extended family.

The following day, my mother called to tell me the news of my dad having a stroke. That was the first sign of his health dwindling. Scissors was right by my side. She held my hand, touched my hair, let me feel sad on her lap, comforting me in a way that made me feel safe. I had never had the inclination that a woman could be a rock for me, and that's when I knew I was falling in love. I hated that it took my father being sick for me to gain that kind of clarity, but it was something I needed to see. I needed to know that my attraction for women wasn't fake or the result of the inherent hypersexuality in me.

Over the course of that year, Scissors became my closest girl-friend and my lover. We spent our weekends going to raves, doing molly, and living our twenties up! Like clockwork, we'd clock out of work and head to the club. Part of the sexiness of our relationship was the stares we'd get that made me feel judged and turned on at the same time. Sometimes, when we would kiss, I would lock eyes with a random person because I knew that we didn't fit the typical lesbian mold. No offense to my masc girls out there! But Scissors and I were the two lipstick lesbians that guys fantasize about, and I began to feel guilty about how much I enjoyed the male gaze when I was around her. Even though, yes, I did find the nights out to be part of the foreplay, my intimacy with her was beautiful. We would hold hands on a long drive without talking. Hold each other at night, locking fingers and facing each other. Sometimes she'd come into the bathroom while I brushed my teeth in the mornings and kiss my neck, attached to me the entire time. Making the first move was what I thought masculinity was, but it just came naturally to us.

The patriarchy had made me feel like a man had to be an initiator when it came to acts of physical affection, which led me to believe that I would be missing that with her. But she was nothing short of romantic. And the sex!! WHEW!! Phenomenal. On a list of best lovers, she's in my top three. And because she'll, without a shadow of a doubt, read this chapter, I refuse to let her know where she's placed in that lineup. Anyway, on to the kinda gayer stuff.

Sex with Scissors was a mixture of passion, learning, and teaching. There are a multitude of ways girls like to fuck . . . but our way was clearly SCISSORING. Like my first experience with a woman, the kissing didn't compare to kisses with men. It made me hornier than any kiss I've had with any man in my life. Maybe it was the softness of the touch on my face, the shyness in who was going to put their tongue where, or the hair my fingers would get wrapped up in. It was like doing something forbidden and right for me, all in the same breath.

Scissors and I would always start with a kiss and roll around the bed for almost an hour before our clothes even came off. We always had sex to the TV light. We'd play MTV, and the late-night music videos would determine what activity came next. I remember one night, Usher's "Nice & Slow" came on, and she got on top of me, grinding while she had her hand on my neck. Suddenly, A$AP Rocky's "Fuckin' Problems" came on, and she said, "AHHHHH SHIT BITCH," and got up to start twerkin'. The playfulness of our sex was what made it so unique. I would laugh for fucking hours at her. She was the perfect mixture of a lover and a friend.

When we finally got out of our homegirl headspace, we became utterly obsessed with pleasing each other. We'd almost argue over who would lick the other's pussy first. I preferred it to be me; it's very difficult for me to receive without giving, even today. My favorite position with her was sixty-nine, a perfect mixture of give-and-take.

I loved to have her pussy in my mouth when I was in the middle of an orgasm, and she knew exactly what I liked. She would always withhold my orgasm from me since, according to her, "You turn into a senior citizen after you cum." Paying close attention to my breath, she knew when I was almost at my peak, and she would change position to get right in between my legs.

See, the act of scissoring is way more about getting the right groove than regular penetration. You have to have the right amount of wetness—not too much because you need the friction, but not too little because your pussy has to glide. Scissors was a fucking super soaker. Sometimes I could just start talking about sex, and she would make me feel the literal pool under her skirt. During sex, it was everywhere.

By the time she would get on top of me, there was always juice trailing from my stomach to my thighs. It was the most amazing feeling ever. The second our pussy lips would touch, she was so LOUD! I would watch her, thinking she may be slightly faking, but I felt it, too.

Now, if you live under a rock and have never heard of scissoring— here we go:

> "Scissoring is a sexual position in which two partners
> sit facing each other and cross their legs so that their
> genitals touch. It's called scissoring because the po-
> sition looks like two scissors crossing each other and
> touching at the base where the blades meet, with the
> legs of each partner imitating the blades of scissors."
> —WebMD[*]

Scissors and I had our exploration with strap-ons, dildos, vibrators, and various toys, but nothing was as pleasurable as our own bodies.

We would top each other, finding new ways to take control. I always sensed that I had much less confidence in bed than Scissors. She felt so natural being with me, and it took me time to get there. When it came to being with men, I always thought I had it all figured out. Truth be told, even though I didn't, I didn't care for their opinion as much. I always had a very "you're just lucky to be here" attitude with any man in my presence, but with women I felt the need to be perfect.

There is no way to explain the amount of pressure I put on myself in my relationship with Scissors. The bond that two women share who have previously dated men and now have each other is quite intense. Scissors was the only relationship I had been in where I hadn't been cheated on. Although unspoken, we were well aware that our trauma lay in deception.

Even though our relationship was strained in a lot of ways, there were so many factors in our dynamic that confused me, and to this day, I wish I had the answers sooner. For instance: Was my relationship with Scissors even real? Whenever I was with men, nobody made me feel like that person was a phase. I was so frustrated with the notion that because she was a woman, she wouldn't be my forever person. I dated her in an era when gay dads were in cartoons. Did people seriously think family was out the window because there were two pussies in the picture?

I always say I want a family, but I wasn't as serious as she was back then. She was way more intentional than me. And to her credit, I'm the one who is now scrolling on her page, wishing that I was a part of her family pictures. The words exchanged during our breakup are foggy to me, but the feelings are memorable. The events of the day were: Airport. Kiss. Club. Dinner. Fight. Car. Fight. House.

Beard Bae and I arrived in Florida to spend time with Scissors and we all headed out to a day party, then dinner. The explosion happened when we got into the car. She was passive-aggressive throughout the day about my feelings for her and implied that I wasn't showing up or giving her enough. I didn't understand where it came from then, but looking back, I see what I did wrong. Although we were only two years apart in age, she was approaching thirty and looking at her life through a lens that I couldn't relate to yet. The crazy thing is, I *did* want everything we discussed. Kids, family, and more importantly, unconditional LOVE. The problem was that I never acted on it. I talked about it, but I never found ways to show her that I was ready to take the steps that she was, even though it's what I eventually wanted.

Maybe I really wasn't ready.

Scissors found her happily ever after. She gave birth to a beautiful baby girl a few years ago and I have finally come to the point where I feel no jealousy in my happiness. On a visit to Orlando, I had the pleasure of meeting her daughter at a café. She was the sweetest and happiest baby. I took pics of them that I gazed at from time to time, wondering if I'd made a mistake. But just because our love didn't result in *us* being the happy family, that doesn't mean we failed. She got *exactly* what she wanted. Seeing her happiness as a mother is exactly what I wanted, and I didn't even know it. Through maturation, I've learned that when you really love someone, their happiness is paramount to you, no matter the outcome for yourself.

I would hate for her to read this, but since you're here, I want to tell you this.

TO SCISSORS:

It is completely unfair that I kept you longer than you knew you should stay. My love for you was wrapped in my love for what you did for me. Many times, you have been a reflection of what I wanted for myself, not necessarily the partner that you deserved.

You are part of my proudest moments in life and my biggest regret. I regret that I had no idea how to love you. And I regret that it took so long to tell you I'm sorry.

You hold a special place in my heart and mind and will forever be there. Thank you for the lessons. Scissors, you taught me how to love.

Patriarchal Bullshit

"If you didn't show up today with HIV, AIDS, or any of them deadly sexually transmitted diseases that'll make you die in two to three weeks, then put your cell phone light in the air. Ladies, if your pussy smell like water, put your cell phone light in the air. Fellas, if you ain't suck a n-gga dick in the parking lot, put your cell phone lights in the air."
—DaBaby (rapper)[1]

Matriarchal Reply

"So much fear is put into female sexuality:
'Bad things will happen to you, you'll get attacked, you'll have diseases, people will take advantage of you.'
Sex is the most human exchange you can have.
You've got to go out there and get your anecdotes."
—Caitlin Moran (BBC)[2]

CAN I PUT IT BACK THERE?

« MANDII B »

WHEN I FIRST started fucking, I believed that if a man wanted to put it in my ass that he was gay—period, point blank. You could not tell me otherwise. My rationale was that if I had this glorious pussy (and I do) that there was no reason he should want to put it in the back door. To me, when it came to heterosexual sex, there were only two acceptable orifices: my vagina and my mouth. I thought of anal sex as something that only gay men did. Looking back, I attribute this blatant misconception to many things, including my youth, lack of sexual education, and flat-out ignorance. While anal sex attitudes among hetero partners have begun to shift, this act still carries some stigma and shame. Growing up, none of my friends or peers were even discussing putting it in the butt. Girls who did have anal sex would only do so because they thought they were still considered a virgin if their pussy wasn't penetrated. Sex scenes in films made it seem like a penis penetrating a vagina was already so painful, so trying to stuff it into an even smaller hole was unappealing as fuck. Let's not even get to the idea of the mess yet (but we will).

Shedding the layers of our ignorance can happen in any area we choose. As we journey through life, our perspectives on sex inevitably transform and evolve in ways that mirror the rest of our development. In the same way our vocabularies expand through conversation and reading, our understanding of sexuality deepens with experience and knowledge. Trial and error, so to speak. Our opinions about sex are not fixed but fluid, influenced by culture, education, personal experiences, and societal norms. In a world where official sex education is often inadequate, many of us find ourselves navigating the complexities of sexuality with incomplete information, leading to misconceptions and uninformed views. This chapter explores how our evolving opinions on sex reflect a broader journey of self-discovery and enlightenment.

If you are Black, you probably already know that our community tends to be extremely homophobic. There is likely a simplistic reason for this: "The Black church, the oldest institution and pillar of the Black community, has historically dictated the community's stance on homosexuality—either you don't talk about it, or you condemn it," says journalist and blogger Lynne d Johnson.[3] If you come from a Caribbean background like me, then you know the conversation around homosexuality reeks of ignorance and hate. In Jamaican culture, being gay has always been completely looked down upon. The homophobia runs very deep. You know how we sing songs as kids that we have no business singing along to? My impressionable mind was shaped by the music I listened to. I remember loving a popular reggae song, "Boom Bye Bye," by Buju Banton. I'd wind my little hips and motion my finger as if it were on the trigger of a gun. Here I was, reciting lyrics that depicted the murdering of gay men.

Buju issued an apology after receiving international backlash from the song's 1992 rerelease, and eventually stopped performing it. The track was also removed from streaming platforms.

Growing up, I had a cousin that we all knew was gay, but we were never introduced to his lovers, romantic partners, or that side of his personal life. It recently dawned on me how difficult this had to be for my cousin. The family didn't speak about it, but he also never led with it. I can only think now about how lonely and frustrating that must have been for him.

Up until the age of thirteen or fourteen I had no idea about almost anything when it came to sex besides "insert penis in vagina." Gender identity and the fluidity of sexuality were not discussed among my family, with my peers, or in school. Sex often centered on pleasuring a man to his climax and, for women, the step of motherhood and reproduction. As we will also discuss in my chapter about abortion, no one gave me a proper sexual education. I didn't have any friends who were openly talking about anal play, either. It literally did not seem like an option for a woman because it wasn't a topic of discussion and wasn't introduced on a mainstream level through movies, TV, or music. To make this shit even more interesting, as of 2024, anal sex (sodomy) is still ILLEGAL in Florida as well as twelve other states. Derived from a legal doctrine known as "church law," sodomy ordinances were passed to stop non-procreative sexuality wherever it might be found.[4] Back to the church stepping in and taking all the fun away.

Raised in Florida, I don't remember knowing very many LGBTQIA+ individuals besides my cousin. There weren't a lot of openly gay men or women around while I was growing up, and in school, I noticed the boys who appeared more feminine, but they didn't label themselves as gay. It wasn't until I moved to Atlanta that

I was introduced to a more prominent LGBTQIA+ community. I got a job working at the Lenox Square mall as a stock manager at Diesel, and this is where I remember seeing it all! I saw the boys with nails longer than mine, shorts shorter than mine, and makeup laid better than mine; though San Francisco is known as the Gay Mecca, Atlanta is the Black Gay Mecca of the United States. (I want to point out that sodomy is illegal in Georgia as well.) Living in Atlanta was also the first time I had to do a "temperature check" with the guys I liked. You could not simply assume that anyone was heterosexual. Throw into the mix that Atlanta was the first place a guy had even mentioned anal sex to me. This only solidified my stupid theory in my young mind.

Here is something that I did not take into consideration before now: Why the fuck was I judging anyone when I, too, found freedom and liberation in exploring my sexual landscape with fluidity and inquisitiveness? According to the National Library of Medicine, studies often link bisexuality with higher levels of sexual fluidity, meaning flexibility in sexual attraction depending on the situation or partner, which could manifest as openness to different sexual practices.[5] So maybe that is part of how I finally made a 180-degree transition and attempted to dismantle the negative connotation around acts that didn't seem to fit the heteronormative confines of sex. I took steps to unlearn some of the mistaken tropes about sexuality, anal sex, and the negative connotations surrounding them, and sought to explore more of how I could experience pleasure. On a more basic level, after learning how to do it, I discovered anal sex is fucking fantastic.

Well, not at first. My first time out, no lube was involved, so it did not go well. I went in open and curious, with just spit and hope. Hoping that he would be gentle and hoping my bootyhole would go back to normal. When I think about it now, I just think, *Ouch*. I was nineteen, and my partner wasn't much older than me. We were both inexperienced muthafuckas really trying to get our freak on. A study done in 2019 by the CDC on Youth Risk Behavior found that 36.7 percent of men and 29.7 percent of women have their first experience with anal sex before the age of twenty.[6] There I go, being another statistic.

I remember breathing heavily as I prepared for my asshole to be stretched wide the fuck open. I lay on my side as he lifted my ass cheek to gain entry. Funnily enough, he had difficulty finding the right hole to penetrate. I remember laughing and telling him "Wrong hole" more times than I would have liked. He moved in every which way and tried several positions to make the entrance of his dick into my asshole more comfortable for the both of us. He continued to transfer spit from his mouth to the tip of his dick to help it slide in better. The constant poking at my hole made this experience less enjoyable than it could have been. When he finally got the tip inside, the pain made this experience hell. I tried to take more and wanted to complete the mission psychologically; however, physically, the pain led me to call it off.

So I understand anal sex can still be terrifying. Especially if you've had the "slip out and accidentally end up in the wrong hole" scenario play out for you. I think most of us have been traumatized by that little slip-up. I want to help those who are considering trying anal or want to give it a go again after a failed attempt.

LUBE! HAVE PLENTY OF IT—I'd recommend lube in most sexual experiences, but using lube during penetrative anal play is a MUST. The vagina produces natural lubrication; the anus, not so much. Water-based and silicone-based lubes are safe to use with condoms; oil-based can damage the latex, so be aware of that. You can also consider desensitizing and numbing lube—however, avoid ATM (ass-to-mouth) action when using this. Your whole tongue and mouth will end up numb! Trust me.

DECIDE WHAT YOU WANT TO TRY—Because guess what? You've got options. There is penis-in-anus, toy-in-anus, oral, or just placing a simple finger or two. It is easiest to receive anal sex when you are relaxed and lying on your back if you're a beginner.

CONDOMS, BECAUSE SEXUAL HEALTH IS #1—You can get sexually transmitted infections via your butt. Unless you and your partner(s) are sexually monogamous and have been tested recently, condoms are always a necessity. And remember, when you go from ass to vagina, a fresh condom is a must! You do NOT want that bacteria to go inside your vagina, as it can lead to vaginal or urinary tract infections.

SLOW AND STEADY—When exploring anal with a partner, you will want to reserve some time for foreplay. Give yourself time to relax. Your rectum is designed to keep feces in with help from a muscle called the anal sphincter. This can make anal a challenge. So take it slow. And remember, if it hurts too much, you call the shots and ask your partner to stop.

POOP, BECAUSE LET'S BE REAL—Alex Hall, an anal sex educator, says it best: "Having anal sex and expecting that there is *never* going to be poop is like going in the pool and expecting not to get wet."* During anal play, the activity takes place in the rectum, which usually doesn't store feces unless a bowel movement is imminent. This makes the likelihood of you pooping on your partner very low. If you've recently pooped and don't have unpredictable bowel conditions like ulcerative colitis, unexpected feces are unlikely. However, some fecal residue might remain, exposing your partner to visible or invisible matter. If you choose to use a douche or enema to clean up, Planned Parenthood has some great tips on their site and recommends that you do so "an hour or 2 before, to help your butt recover from any potential irritation."[8]

If I haven't scared you off by mentioning poop, let's move on to the first time that I experienced anal penetration that I genuinely fucking enjoyed.

I had tried it with partners over the years and it was something cool to do, but I wasn't begging for it. That all changed with this guy who still holds a Top 3 ranking in the bedroom for me. On the podcast, he is referenced as 24/7. This became his nickname because he could literally get this pussy 24/7. I would leave my homegirls for the dick. I would set my alarm for all hours of the night so I didn't miss his late-night booty calls. Early on, I was even paying for his cab to come to the Bronx from Harlem to fuck me. I wanted it whenever and wherever, so the nickname felt fitting. He had a hold on me like few other people ever have or ever will. I don't know what made me tell him that I wanted him to fuck me in the ass that night, but I did. I wanted to do anything and everything with him, so I guess asking for anal was a natural progression in our sexual escapades. While we had attempted it a few times before, his dick was just so massive, and maybe I wasn't relaxed enough; it just never seemed to fit. I announced to him over the phone that tonight was the night he was going to fuck me in the ass and that I promised to take it all. I was determined.

24/7 kept his life and his extracurricular activities separate from our rendezvous. He had family staying at his house, so he had a room booked at the DoubleTree in New Jersey across the George Washington Bridge. This was an early night for us because he left the studio at 2 a.m. instead of 4. I met him in the room and immediately worried about making a mess of those clean white sheets on the king-sized bed. We had a routine: we would talk a bit; he would ask me if I wanted a drink; and he would smoke a blunt. I didn't really smoke much because it messed up my voice, but I used to love to suck his big ol' dick while he smoked. The image of him watching me while billows of smoke escaped his lips still turns me on.

I beat him to the room that evening and placed everything in arm's reach. I dug into my purse and hid the lube under my pillow so there wouldn't be any awkward moments searching for it. I was always ready for him; my pussy was leaking before we even started. We fucked first, and then he went to go back into my pussy again, and I said, "No. I want what I asked for." He took me down to the bottom of the bed; looking back, I wonder if this is why it felt so good. Positions do matter when it comes to anal, so switch it up. I stayed on my back and pulled the lube out from under my pillow. As I lay at the bottom of the bed with the lube right next to me, I went back to sucking his dick to be sure it was as hard as I knew it could get.

Once he was rock solid, I rubbed the lube all over his throbbing member and around my asshole. His dick slid right in, and the only word that I can think of to describe this experience is "euphoria." I was like, *What is going on? This is amazing!* I felt like I was squirting from my ass, cumming in a way I had never experienced before. He leaned over me while he was fucking me in my ass, and he started whispering all this sexy and nasty shit to me. My pussy was pulsing. I didn't understand what was happening. I was like, *Why is this so good in this hole?* And then I worried, *There is no way this bed is not going to be a fucking mess.* I had cum so hard that I was just sure a flood of shit would be left on the sheets. I was so scared to look down at the bed when we finished. I thought I'd had the literal shit fucked out of me, but I hadn't. My beautiful body was like, *I got you, baby.*

We both came in ecstasy as I allowed him to fuck my ass like it was my pussy. Luckily for me, one round was never enough for us. He was ready to go again. We fucked until he climaxed into the condom in my asshole a second time, and I came for what felt like the millionth time that night. I couldn't stop shaking and cumming. It is essential for me to reiterate that this was the most relaxed I'd ever been during anal, so I know that played an important role in the way this experience went. I had asked for it. I'd mentally prepared myself to desire it and prepped my mind to allow the muscles in my body to fuckin' relax! It didn't hurt that he'd whispered, "This feels so good; let me stay here, please." I obliged.

I have a running joke that I allow and request anal just once a quarter. I will be very real and let you know that the twenty-four hours following anal sex, you'll feel anxious about shit just falling right out of you. Over time, I have also learned to use other tools like dilators and butt plugs. I have evolved enough to understand that anything done between a man and a woman is indeed heterosexual sex. We can explore our bodies in so many ways if we allow ourselves to. Once we remove the ignorance and preconceived notions of what things are "bad" or "wrong" in sex, we can naturally reach heights of pleasure that we may have once thought were impossible. This has allowed me to explore sexuality in ways that I had never imagined.

BUT WAIT, THERE'S MORE . . .

Ironically, the woman who once thought that if a man wanted to fuck her in the ass it meant he was gay has no shame about how much she likes to play with a man's ass today. Now that you have stayed with me this far, I will tell you how my nickname Peg Thee Stallion came into existence. And I think I would be doing a goddamn disservice to you and myself if I didn't share this. When it comes to my role with men and anal play, I have graduated from using my tongue, to using my finger, to discovering one of my favorite pastimes: pegging. For those of you who don't know, pegging is an anal sex act that usually involves a cis woman penetrating a man's anus with a strap-on dildo.

Let me share the first time I ever did this with a man. It was his first time as well. He had one rule: he wanted us to use a dildo that did not look like a dick. Thinking back, for a straight man who had never felt comfortable enough to try this before, this request certainly made sense. I went to the sex shop and bought a prostate dildo that had a curved tip, and I let the lady there know that I planned to use it on a man. She told me that the curve should always face his belly button; if he was on his back, it should be facing up, and if he was on his knees, it should face down. It was so hard and stiff, and although I would have preferred a brown, veiny, natural-looking dildo, I wanted to make my partner as comfortable as possible. The chosen dildo didn't even come in flesh-tone colors, so I purchased it in purple.

Hell, at the time I wasn't a pro myself, so there were many things I wish I knew better. I only knew that I had to be very gentle and use a lot of lube. In my Keith Lee voice, I will say I rate my first experience with pegging a 5.5 out of 10. The dildo was extremely hard and uncomfortable, and it took me a while to find a position that worked with our height difference.

After this experience, it was so much fun to exchange notes. We both agreed that we needed a softer dildo, and he said that the next purchase would be a more lifelike dildo. He didn't want it too thick, and we still decided it wouldn't be flesh-toned so as not to emulate an actual dick. This is probably the beginning of one of the best things to happen during my sexual journey. I began to communicate not only before sex, but also after.

Here are a few pointers to ensure new experiences in the bedroom with your partner don't result in trauma:

BEGIN WITH AFFIRMATIONS—Let your partner know how much you enjoyed yourself and how grateful you are to have had this exchange with them.

DON'T BE AFRAID TO SAY WHAT YOU DIDN'T ENJOY—If something was not enjoyable, you must express this (e.g., "Babe, I know we tried something new with the pillowcase last night, but I didn't really enjoy it. Let's not do that again.").

REMOVE YOUR EGO—When communicating about the intimacy of sex and what you liked and did not like, be open to receiving criticism. What is good for one person might not be for the next.

TAKE IT OUT OF THE BEDROOM—You don't want to build up anxiety with your partner that every time you get into bed, there will be a lecture or deep convo of some sort. Make talking about sex without having sex a regular thing in your relationship.

One of the greatest feelings I have around pegging in particular is the trust that I have to build with my partners, who have granted me access to their bootyholes. As discussed before, there are stigmas around anal sex within our community and its direct link to homophobia: a man's asshole is the gateway to gay, and once you're gay, then you are damned to hell for eternity. This is what the church has ingrained in so many of us. I would have to reassure my partner that if he was doing this with me, a woman, he was not gay. I find joy in being with someone who can remove shame and fear and genuinely enjoy consensual, kinky fun! In a sexually liberated era, I love that, as women, we can embrace our sexuality and live a little more loud in the open, and I want our Black brothers to be able to do the same.

I was also into watching gay porn at this time, and I wanted to be a part of that world (as much as any woman can). As cell phones became more advanced, the ease of porn at my fingertips allowed me to stumble across far more genres of sex than I had been privy to previously. I found a gay male porn scene where both men were beautifully chiseled, they moaned with enjoyment, and they took their time. It intrigued me. I didn't have to sit through a bad weave job or look at a man in Timberland boots completely obliterating a pussy. Porn between two men seemed more passionate and intentional. It was a way I hadn't seen men before. I saw men having big orgasms from having their prostates milked, and maybe it was my competitive nature, but I wanted to please a man in the same fashion. Though my first time wasn't perfect, I dusted myself off and tried again with someone else.

I had been talking to this guy I had met on Instagram for years. He played ball overseas, and during those months while he was away, we would spend hours chatting on the phone about everything—the difference in culture where he was, the foods, and, of course, sex. We would send each other nudes and share porn. As I mentioned, communicating wants and needs, desires and fantasies, with a prospective lover is crucial. I know one-night stands can be exciting, and sometimes you're let down after a massive buildup of talking, but I love to get into how kinky a muthafucka can be and what possible adventures we could have in the bedroom. We found ourselves talking about butt play, and to my surprise and excitement, he expressed an interest in trying out pegging. He had gotten his ass eaten and been penetrated by one finger, but at this time, he hadn't been bent over and strapped. We were exhilarated at the thought, and he even went so far as to prepare himself for me. He went to the sex store and purchased the tiniest dildo I had ever seen. It looked to be the size of a damn thumb, but I genuinely appreciated his efforts and the baby steps to opening that thang up for me.

He had a twelve-hour layover on his way back home. I got us a room in Times Square, where I was working. We planned to have dinner, visit a sex store, and then explore a sex club together. Dinner was hilarious because our dumb asses chose a steak house, but we both knew we didn't want shitty asses for our late-night escapades. Red meat wouldn't be a smart choice, nor the dairy-filled potatoes or macaroni. We indulged in drinks and kept dinner light.

We left the restaurant and walked a few blocks to a sex store situated next to a liquor store. Our giddiness was undeniable. Were we really about to fuckin' do this? We headed to the section with the harnesses and dildos. I got a harness that could securely and comfortably fit my thick thighs. We then chose to buy two dildos—one medium-sized and one a little larger. Both were brown, veiny, natural dick-looking dildos. We got lube and poppers at the counter and then headed to the liquor store to cop a bottle of tequila for the room. We were too excited. We showered and got ready for the club, took multiple shots, made out, and even got a quickie in. At one point, I was lying on the bed and he walked over and sat on my big toe. This muthafucka let me toe fuck his ass!

This isn't a chapter about the sex club, but just know he fucked me DOWN in front of strangers that evening, and we ended the night in a shower with two other couples. The six of us licked and sucked one another while the rest of the attendees watched in awe. Needless to say, our horny meters were through the damn roof by the time we got back to the room. We hadn't brought any of the toys to the sex club because we wanted to enjoy this moment in private.

He threw me on the bed and kissed me while undressing me at the same time. His kisses were followed by "thank yous" as he expressed how grateful he was to have had his first sex club experience. His dick was throbbing at attention for the third time that night. He was ready to go! My pussy leaking from all the previous excitement made it easy for his dick to slide right in me. As he fucked me, I let him know how good I'd be fucking him in exchange. "You ready for me to open up that tight little ass?" He moaned loud and thrust his dick even harder inside of me. "I'm gonna fuck that ass so good and make you my slut. You gonna be my good little slut?" He let out a sexy "YES!" As he reached across to the end table to grab the lube and poppers, he began to mentally prepare. I went to the foot of the bed, put on my harness, and grabbed the smaller dildo of the two. He directed me to get the bigger one. A mischievous smile came across my face.

He assumed the position on all fours. I massaged his lower back while I ate his ass. I wanted to be sure he was relaxed and that we didn't rush. He sniffed the poppers, and I replaced my saliva on his ass with the lube we had purchased. We had officially entered our own premeditated porn scene. Before I got behind him, I told him to suck my strap and get it wet. Although I also planned to add lube, seeing him sucking the dildo he selected was fuckin' hot! I stood up and assumed a frog position to insert my dick into his ass—once I have a dick in a harness, it becomes MY DICK.

I took my time. I went slow. I spoke affirmations to him as I slid inside and opened him up. "You're being such a good boy. Open that tight hole for me, baby." I was leaking down my fucking leg! The sight of this beautifully tatted 6'6" man taking my brown, veiny, natural-looking dildo drove me crazy. He went from being on all fours to lying on his back, holding his long legs in the air as I penetrated him in a missionary position. We fucked each other until the early morning! He even changed his flight to leave three hours later than initially planned so we could keep going. This was, by far, the sexiest, kinkiest, most fun evening of sex and orgasms.

In sharing how far I have come and how much my point of view on anal sex and play has changed, I am asking you to keep an open mind as well. We have a lot of deprogramming to do, which is essential for a healthy sex life. Figuring out what to do and how to do it is actually the easiest part of the process. It's often said that good sex is 80 percent mental and only 20 percent physical for women. So for many of us, we have to get out of our damn heads. You can start with trying something simple that you have always wanted to explore. I'm not asking you to go out and buy a harness, but if you want to, I see you, sister! Your next step can be as easy as testing a new position, having sex in a new place (even just a different space in your home), watching a specific type of porn, or getting a new toy. There are no hard and fast rules. The only rule is to keep trying new things and discovering new ways to find pleasure for you and your partner.

Patriarchal Bullshit

"Women are meant to be loved, not to be understood."
—Oscar Wilde (author of *Lord Arthur Savile's Crime and Other Stories*)[1]

Matriarchal Reply

"No one can make you feel inferior without your consent."
—Eleanor Roosevelt (former First Lady of the United States)[2]

IS PROTECTION EVEN PLEASURABLE?

« WEEZYWTF »

SAFETY WITHIN YOUR body, safety in your community, safety of the heart—this is the trifecta of protection. It might not sound as exciting as the wild stories you've read so far, but believe me, this is the chapter you *need*. This isn't the climax you may have seen coming for this section (no pun intended), but understanding safety is one of the most important lessons in my journey.

Consider this your road map to ensuring you take care of your vehicle, have a healthy relationship with your crew, and never end up with another tragic ex. Well, I can't promise the last one; if I could, Mandii and I would be out of the podcast game. But you will learn to set your boundaries.

LITERAL SAFETY

Let's start by acknowledging that you've probably heard the standard safety spiel a thousand times: share your location, carry pepper spray, and walk with your keys between your fingers like a mini-Wolverine.

Be ready to jack an asshole as you traverse that lonely subway tunnel. God help us all!

When it comes to sex, the safety conversation is generally about barrier methods like condoms and dental dams. But somehow, we rarely discuss literal physical safety, so I have decided that this is an excellent time to share my personal ONE-NIGHT STAND RULES:

LOCATION, LOCATION: This goes beyond just turning on my location and sharing with friends. I also let him KNOW a friend knows my location.

I always have a friend call me, and I answer with:

Me: "Hey, girl, I gotta go. Call you in the morning. . . . Oh, sure, I can do that tomorrow. I'm just here around 46th and 8th, so I'm not too far from you. . . . Yes, I am with {IN-SERT THEIR NAME}. Things obviously went well, haha okay, gotta go now, sis, bye!"

I always make sure the person I'm with knows that someone else is very aware of who they are and where I am.

Actually, nine times out of ten when I'm comfortable with some-one, I eventually share my lie with my date, and they pass this safety gem on to their homegirls.

I ASK MYSELF HOW I FEEL: I don't care if I am already in his bed and in my underwear. If the vibe is off, the vibe is off. HELL YES is the only response I want to give myself and my partner when engaging in sex for the first time, and I have made that promise so that I never have to feel bad about the decision the next day.

HARD LIMITS: Even if the person I'm about to sleep with is in the middle of taking my clothes off, I'm having a sexy conversation about how I need to be treated during sex. I have found in my chats with close girlfriends that they seem to feel like it's awkward to list their desires or turn-offs with someone they have just met. If you are one of these people, here are two examples of what that conversation can sound like:

"I can't wait to fuck you, but I really want you to please me. I'm the most turned on when I'm gripped by my ass and my waist, but never my neck. No choking tonight, please."

"Just to let you know, I love being talked to; I just don't like rough or dirty talk. But when you slide inside of me and find out how good my pussy is gripping, please tell me that!"

As I log the final piece of how to keep yourself safe . . . out of all the embarrassing shit I've already disclosed so far in the book, it would be wrong of me to not talk about every woman's greatest nightmare, aka A STANK PUSSY.

SEXUAL HEALTH SAFETY

In a strange way, even though we're overloaded with conversations surrounding caring for our body and health, advice tends to go in one ear and out the other. Exchanging or asking for someone's STD results sounds good until you think about doing it, and the thing that stops you . . . it's just too awkward. I've tended to sweep uncomfortable conversations under the rug, and I pay for it in the end.

Even if it isn't a sexually transmitted disease, there's still the possibility of that great nightmare most commonly known as bacterial vaginosis. It has to be the most excruciating hell known to womankind.

"Bacterial vaginosis (BV) is a common vaginal infection that happens when some normal bacteria that live in your vagina overgrow, causing a bacterial imbalance. Symptoms include an off-white or gray vaginal discharge that smells 'fishy.' BV is easily treatable with antibiotics from a healthcare provider."[3]

You can get BV in many ways, including simply going for a swim. More commonly in adults, it's from unprotected sex. There's no real way to protect yourself 100 percent from STIs in oral or non-penetrative sex. The only way to do that would be to test ahead of time. I never thought my kinks could take my body from healthy to turmoil, but I've had to atone for my actions a time or three for the sexiest way I receive pleasure.

I'm a total cum slut. I have said more than a hundred times on our show how much I enjoy watching bukkake porn. I honestly don't even know where this obsession came from. Having it in my mouth, having it on my skin, watching it drip out of a dick; even the pre-cum when it's not fully white yet; the dribbling of it back onto the dick, letting it drip out of my mouth and fall onto my chest; maybe cum swapping in a threesome, maybe snowballing with him . . . OH THE ENDLESS POSSIBILITIES OF CUM!

My ultimate favorite, which is the creampie, is literally the largest threat to the health of my vagina.

With my current partner, we did have a few condomless mistakes before trading results, but once we did . . . THE SEX LIFE TURNED UP, HUN. As you know, I'm a girl who's kinda gay . . . but this is the one thing I get excited about when being in a relationship with a man. There is no sexier dirty talk than being able to ask someone to cum inside of you. But once it's in there, I'd equate the feeling of being a cum dump to that of a man with post-nut clarity.

Like, seriously, what the fuckkk was I thinking? Not only do I have thirty days to wait and make sure I'm not pregnant, but two or three days later, the SMELL hits. Maybe it's a trip to the bathroom. You pull your panties down and hope that maybe you didn't drink enough water. Perhaps it happens at the gym: you get off that treadmill and hope you just sweat too much.

Nah, girl. It's BV.

Listen, I'm no doctor, but I'm going to give you my best tips to keep your vaginal health intact.

PEE AFTER SEX—Always pee it out and clean yourself off before going back to bed.

REGULARLY TAKE PROBIOTICS—My personal fave is RAW Probiotics Vaginal Care by Garden of Life.

DON'T DOUCHE!—This removes all the good bacteria you need to prevent infection. You may be trying to mask a scent, but you'll only make things worse.

The worst part of ending up with BV or some other sort of pussy issue is that everyone will think you're gross because of the smell. It's the most embarrassing thing a partner could tell you, the most shameful conversation to have with a doctor, and in the mix of trying to find ways of keeping your body safe, you realize . . . you don't have a safe space for this! It should be your friends, but friends aren't supposed to be that involved in your business . . . or are they?

COMMUNAL SAFETY

As the years go by, I've grown more grounded in the fact that friends are your chosen family. Let's be honest—everyone's family is fucked up. There's most likely someone in the bloodline who's an alcoholic, who has an addiction, who's always asking you for money, or who you wouldn't choose to spend your holidays with. But the strangers we collect and choose to keep on this crazy journey called life? *That's* your real family.

When you're a baby, your safety net is your parents. But when you're grown, who the hell is there to wipe your tears? Sure, there's therapy, but let's be real—they're getting paid. What we need is COMMUNITY. I watched this documentary on Netflix called *Live to 100: Secrets of the Blue Zones*, and it showed people who live to one hundred years old and beyond. Across Japan, California, Sardinia, Costa Rica, and Singapore, they all had one thing in common: community.

I don't know about you, but I'm tired of the whole "you don't need anybody but yourself" narrative. Sure, you don't need toxic people, but genuine friendship and care? That's what holds you down when life gets heavy.

Each birthday tags on another +1, and the friendships become –1. I'll never forget when my friend Emilie said, "At this age, the friends you have right now are the ones who will be consoling you when your parents die." That hit me like a ton of bricks. It made me realize I didn't want to keep any more surface-level friendships. There's just no more space in my life for people who don't accept me, who talk behind my back, or who think my sexuality is all about the male gaze. Even in my relationship with Scissors, I heard, "She's just doing this because dudes think it's sexy." I am so absolutely DONE with friends who low-key hate me!

The key to friendship is to find people who fully accept you as their chosen family. Luckily for me, the ones I've got have done just that.

Me: "Shit, I fucked him last night."
Friend: "WEEZY! But didn't you fuck his homeboy???"
Me: "I knoooowwwwww, I knowwwwwwwww!!!"
Friend: "Well, was it fun?"

THIS IS THE ONLY TYPE OF ENERGY I WANT.

The nonjudgmental friend isn't merely the one who's just as much of a dirty little demon as you are. No, this vibe comes from someone who's fully embraced the person they are—someone who can appreciate your vulnerability and radical authenticity while letting their love for you shine.

For me, that's Venny and Brianda—the devil and angel on my shoulders.

THE DEVIL ON YOUR SHOULDER, AKA "THE CHEERLEADER"

Venny! Where do I even start with this friendship? He's my best friend, my ride-or-die, the one friend I celebrate anniversaries with. We've got matching tattoos—two of them—and he's more family to me than just a friend. Gay, Haitian, and my literal twin. We first met at EDC in New York City around 2010; ever since then, we've been inseparable. Now, he's checked me before about calling him my "gay bestie" (because it reduces him to his sexuality), and I totally get that. But honestly, in the beginning, I thought that was why we had this crazy magnetic connection. His gayness was something I connected with so deeply, especially since I was in the process of figuring out my own.

After Venny and I fell in love at that first music festival, we met up again at Ultra in Miami, and by the third time we hung out, we were living together. My friendship with Venny defined my early twenties. I mean, I hadn't even slept with a white guy before Venny swiped him right for me while we were chilling in bed.

My level of possession over Venny is honestly insane. If his own mother hadn't given birth to him, I'd probably be jealous of how much attention he gives her—but whatever, it's fine. I gained the brother I was always supposed to have with this friendship—a brother encouraging me to sleep with as many people as possible before getting married.

The thing about meeting the devil on your shoulder is that they make all the "shameful" things you once questioned feel normal. It's this wide-open space for freedom and exploration in conversation. A place where you can confess your dirtiest, darkest thoughts and know that instead of judgment, you'll be met with laughter and re-latability.

Your devil friend will *never* let you sulk over something you did last night. They'll always remind you that your choices—no matter how wild—are shaping who you'll become. (Even the choice to make Venny lie to my date about me being sick while I was getting my back blown out down the hall.) If you ever need someone to talk you *out* of something . . . don't call this friend.

They'll always steer you toward fun, freedom, and a little bit of MISCHIEF.

THE ANGEL, AKA "THE RATIONAL ONE"

Brianda! What can I say about this absolute sweetheart? Though our friendship only began in 2019, I hold it in such high regard. I first met her on the set of her podcast at the time, *Super Trip Talk*, which was all about psychedelics and religion. After vibing with her for an hour, I invited Brianda to an event at House of Yes in Brooklyn. It's a club known for wild costumes, performances, and nonstop dancing, so I figured, as a Brooklyn girl herself, she'd seen it all before.

Well, let's say the night got weird fast. There was some wild burlesque action, a magician eating fake blood, and within twenty minutes, someone was pouring candle wax over my chest like it was supposed to be a pearl necklace. Poor Brianda looked like she was ready to break out in prayer for all the "witchcraft" happening around her. Meanwhile, I thought, *Isn't this just a typical Wednesday night in Bushwick?*

Despite the craziness of that night, my friendship with Brianda kept growing, and to my surprise, it's been entirely free of judgment.

I found myself calling Brianda often for advice about issues in my non-monogamous relationship at the time—something she would *never* consider for herself, but she was open-minded enough to listen. That's when I realized stereotypes are complete bullshit. The "angel" in your life feels like a warm hug, a safe space where you can be emotionally vulnerable without fear of judgment.

This friend could be in bed with their husband, taking their kids to school, or in the middle of work—it doesn't matter. They will always make time to listen and respond in a way that doesn't make you feel small or judged. Brianda didn't need to have personal experience to empathize and help me navigate that one threesome where I got jealous because the other girl sucked my ex's dick better!

I started to pick up a lot of bad habits after my relationship with an ex, especially when I began missing the intimacy. Honestly, I couldn't care less about that "single and loving it" hype when I'm deep in my breakup feelings. The real excitement of being single only hits when you've forgiven them—and yourself. My go-to coping mechanisms were drinking, drugs, and food benders, which, let's be honest, are a common aftermath of breakups no matter where you're from or what gender you are.

It's like an actual stage of grieving.

"There's so many fish in the sea."

"You're better off alone."

WHERE ARE THE FISH? AND I'M BORED AS HELL ALONE.

Your angel friend may not always be down for a wild night out when you need to escape the world, but they will find a way to ground you and help bring you peace. Brianda is that for me. She actively listened to my pain, talked sense into me about what I truly deserved, and handled my feelings with so much care.

Even in moments when I felt like I might relapse and go back to him, she stayed nonjudgmental and encouraged me to embrace a healthier phase of life ahead. As agnostic as I am, my angel friend sometimes prays with me, sometimes without me, but always *for* me. It's not about how often we see each other, but it's always worth it when we do.

Finding community as an adult isn't the easiest thing, but if you have friends, remember this: sometimes we get so wrapped up in our own lives that we forget who might need us the most. Consider this a reminder to respond to that unanswered text about lunch, set up a FaceTime catch-up, or share a meme to reconnect with someone you care about but haven't given much attention to lately. Community is about belonging, having a purpose, and being able to turn to a safe place when times get tough.

Here's how you know you've found your people:

YOU CAN BE 100 PERCENT YOU—No filter, no edits. They love you for who you are, even the messy parts.

THEY SHOW UP, PERIOD—Whether for the big life stuff or just to chill when you're feeling low, your people are always down, even when life gets wild.

ZERO JUDGMENT—You can share your craziest thoughts or biggest mistakes without worrying about side-eye. It's all love.

THEY KEEP IT REAL WITH YOU—Your people won't let you play yourself. They'll call you out when needed but always have your back.

THEY HYPE YOU UP—Your wins are *their* wins. No shade, no competition—just pure celebration for your glow-up.

THEY VIBE WITH YOU ON EVERY LEVEL—Whether it's a night out turning up or a deep convo about life, they match your energy.

THEY FEEL LIKE HOME—Being with them just feels right. There's no need to pretend; you're safe, seen, and understood.

THEY STICK AROUND, EVEN WHEN THINGS GET MESSY—They've seen your worst and still choose to stay. They're down to ride through the rough patches with you.

YOU'RE LEVELING UP TOGETHER—Your people push you to grow, and they're right there growing with you. The bond just gets stronger.

TIME AND DISTANCE DON'T MATTER—Even if you haven't seen them in a minute, the connection is still tight. You pick up like nothing's changed.

EMOTIONAL SAFETY

There are plenty of men I've completely fucked and forgotten, men I've shed tears over—no surprise there. Women, though? Not so much. And honestly, that's because many women seem to crave transparency. Some days, I wish I could reject how much I love dick because being a lesbian seems like it'd be so much easier on the heart. Not because women are soft, but because, in my experience, they've had higher emotional intelligence.

It's not that men don't have feelings—of course they do! But the way they process and communicate those feelings? That's the world's greatest mystery. It's like trying to crack a code that doesn't exist.

This next section isn't about solving that mystery, though. It's about helping you navigate your own journey and learn how to protect your heart by setting boundaries.

This is easier said than done, because when the sex is good, all the rules go out the window. And morality? Gone. That's the real problem—we make our most irrational decisions when we're lonely or horny. (I don't even need an Ivy League study to back that up.) "Boundaries" gets thrown around as a buzzword, but what does it really look like when you put them into action and practice them?

BOUNDARIES WITH PARTNERS

PHASE 1: Weezy meets a new guy. Plans are set, but new guy shows up twenty minutes late. Weezy decides to wait. When he finally arrives, she greets him and immediately tells him that lateness is a major sore spot for her and something she won't tolerate.

PHASE 2: Weezy fucks the new guy. Damn, the dick is *good*. Boundaries? What boundaries? Memory loss kicks in.

PHASE 3: Weezy has been hooking up with this guy for about a month. They plan to meet for drinks at 7 p.m. By 7:11, he's still not there—Weezy dips.

Now, this may sound basic, but we all tend to overlook the boundaries we've failed to set when we start complaining about how people treat us. Are they just treating us the way we *allow* them to? As simple as lateness may seem to some, it can feel like a major form of disrespect to others.

We can't expect people to guess what's acceptable—we must *express* our needs. I firmly believe that real change in a relationship only happens when those needs are communicated, not when they're left as some kind of guessing game.

BOUNDARIES WITH YOURSELF

Weezy experiences painful heartbreak. She replays everything that went wrong, torturing herself over why she stayed. She vents about the same things over and over on the phone with friends, hoping that talking it through will make it all click. She swears to herself she'll never date "someone like that" again.

But what does that vow *really* look like? How do you hold yourself to a promise when it's only for you?

For me, that vow is fundamental when it's written down—not in the Notes app, but with actual pen and paper. It's the most basic form of catharsis, but getting it all out in writing is how I process things. I jot down every raw emotion I felt, every red flag I ignored, and exactly how the pain hit me.

One of my vows is scribbled on the back of a Con Edison bill, tucked away in a stack of old diaries:

> I will never let another human being make me feel this low again. *Low.* I hate him. Hate this feeling. Hate how I feel now. How do I even have the power to write this? I have no power. How can I? It's not just about how it feels; it's about what I'd never allow someone else to feel.

> I would never tell someone to stay. When *redacted* lies to me, it's so easy. It's easy because it's second nature for him, and my second nature is to trust. I *must* trust myself first. Trust yourself. Trust yourself. Trust

yourself. Why don't I trust that I'll be okay before I
trust my heart with him?

Writing it down makes it real, something I can return to when
I feel myself slipping. It reminds me that the only person I need to
trust is myself.

I AM BETTER THAN *REDACTED*.

I AM GOING TO FINALLY LEAVE *REDACTED*.

I AM GOING TO LEAVE HIM WITHIN THE NEXT 7 DAYS AND

PURSUE MY OWN HAPPINESS.

I AM HAPPY

I AM JOY

I AM LOVE

I cried so hard when I wrote it that the ink blurred from the tear-
drops, smudging the words across the page. But honestly, I *needed*
to see that. Even now, just typing it out for the world to see has me
in tears. I needed to capture my desperation on that page—to me-
morialize my lowest moment in a way that feels real and tangible—
because the truth is, as time goes on, I tend to forget.

But here's the thing: never let yourself forget what you've been
through as time passes. Acknowledging our pain is the key to setting
boundaries and sticking to them. Forgetting it doesn't help.

Understanding that just because something *could* be worse
doesn't mean it *can't* get better is powerful.

Life *is* better than whatever bad situation you're in right now.

And life alone? It's more fulfilling than being stuck in incompatibility.

Here are some tangible ways to protect yourself from heartbreak:

SET YOUR BOUNDARIES AND STICK TO 'EM—Lay it all out from the jump—what you need and what you won't tolerate—and make sure you hold yourself to those standards. Boundaries are your armor.

LISTEN TO YOUR GUT—If something feels off, trust that vibe. Your intuition is your built-in radar—don't ignore it.

SLOW YOUR ROLL—Don't rush into something just because it feels good. Take your time, get to know the person, and make sure they're really on your level.

PUT YOURSELF FIRST—Self-love is the foundation. When you know your worth, you won't let anyone treat you with less than you deserve.

KEEP IT 100 WITH YOUR FEELINGS—Say what you mean and mean what you say. Don't hold back on the real talk, even when it's hard. Clear communication prevents messy misunderstandings.

DON'T SELL OUT YOUR VALUES—Stay true to who you are and your beliefs. Don't twist yourself up to fit into someone else's world.

KEEP YOUR SQUAD CLOSE—Back to your community above! Don't lose touch with your friends just because you're in a relationship. Your crew will keep you grounded and remind you of your worth.

BE COOL WITH BEING SOLO—Learn to love your own company. When you're good at being alone, you won't settle for less just to avoid loneliness.

KNOW WHEN TO BOUNCE—Recognize when the situation ain't serving you anymore. Have the strength to walk away before you lose yourself in it.

LEARN FROM YOUR PAST—Heartbreak is a lesson. Reflect on

your past relationships and the red flags you missed so you don't repeat the same mistakes.

Ultimately, safety—whether in your body, community, heart, or love relationships—comes down to knowing yourself and standing firm in what you deserve. The people who truly belong in your life will honor your boundaries and celebrate your growth, not tear it down. This chapter may not have been the wildest ride. Still, it's about the essential lessons: prioritize your emotional, physical, and mental well-being; hold on to your chosen family; and always choose the love that lifts you up, because the real adventure in life is finding the people who make you feel safe enough to be your most authentic self.

PAIN

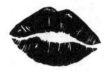

Without pain we could never know pleasure.

When we acknowledge and face our pain, we can create space
for healing and growth. Embracing and growing through pain
allows us to uncover our hidden strengths. This can foster a
more profound sense of self and a greater capacity for resilience.
Through suffering, we can open ourselves to transformation.
Then we can find meaning in even the most challenging experiences.

Surviving painful experiences is where we often learn how to heal
and progress. And that is the entire fucking point of this life.

Patriarchal Bullshit
"It is the law of nature that woman should
be held under the dominance of man."
—Confucius (Chinese philosopher)[1]

Matriarchal Reply
"I am sensual and very physical. I'm very erotic.
But my sexuality exists on a sort of a fantasy level."
—Donna Summer (singer and iconic disco queen)[2]

CAN I PUT
YOUR PENIS IN
A CAGE?

« MANDII B »

SEXUAL ORIENTATION AND the way we experience sex through-out our life is a complex and multifaceted aspect of human identity influenced by three main factors—psychological, biological, and environmental.[3] Factors such as personality traits and life experiences can influence what physical characteristics a person might seek in a partner or their chances to try new things. For example, extroverts naturally socialize and engage more, while introverts may find it difficult to create an atmosphere conducive to engaging in sex with other people. So, as you might expect, a large study of university students in West Germany found that extroverts have more sex than introverts. Biological factors such as genetics and hormones in the womb may impact a person's sexual orientation. You heard that right! You can actually be born gay! Lastly, environmental factors such as culture, familial upbringing, and social norms play, in my opinion, the most significant role in shaping someone's sexual orientation.

For example, a person who grows up in a small town with a strong religious background will have a much different sexual path than that of a person who grows up in a major city with liberal family values. While saying that seems equivalent to saying water is wet, we often don't take the time to consider how these things impact our sexual journeys. My environment absolutely shaped how I navigated my sexuality. Growing up in Florida with a Caribbean family influenced my lack of sexual education and ignorance around same-sex relationships. Being in Atlanta in my later adolescence opened my mind to queer identity. However, the greatest impact on my overall journey, by far, was moving to the city that never sleeps, New York City!

When I decided to move to NYC from the South, I'd already envisioned how I would meet the love of my life. Every way that I wanted to fall in love and enjoy time with my partner mirrored a romantic film. I'd visualized myself rain-soaked, in an alleyway, lip-locked with my soulmate like the kiss between Audrey Hepburn and George Peppard in *Breakfast at Tiffany's*. I even imagined working a low-paying job and being swept off my feet by a wealthy politician like Jennifer Lopez's character in *Maid in Manhattan*. And though it highlighted the ups and downs of dating, I'd be irresponsible not to mention the impact of *Sex and the City* and what I thought my dating life would look like once I got here. Coining myself as the Samantha Jones of my crew, I was ready to sleep with Wilhelmina models and artists I met at the most random events and nonchalantly kick them to the curb as if they didn't matter. I had so many ideas about how my love life would transform. However, New York blessed me with something I had never considered would be pivotal to my actual sexual journey—community.

One random Thursday afternoon, I got a text from a friend who was visiting New York for work. This friend, King Noire, is a renowned and well-endowed sex worker who owns his own company, Royal Fetish Films, for which he and his wife engage in acts of lovely filth. We had plans to link up on the Lower East Side for drinks and small bites. We found ourselves at Verlaine, a little Thai restaurant with $5 martinis for happy hour (now $8 due to inflation). King informed me that his friend, Troy, would be joining us. He let me know that they had plans later that evening. I'm always down to meet new people, so I told him, "The more, the merrier!"

We had the chance to catch up on all the new things in our lives before Troy joined us. I saw an olive-skinned woman with short gray hair and a warm smile approach the table. Her voice was soft, but when she spoke to King, she talked with conviction and dominance. It wasn't until about forty-five minutes into drinks and food that they told me about their relationship. Troy owned a sex dungeon in Chelsea and was teaching King Noire how to properly use flogging tools and leather whips with partners. My jaw almost dropped to the floor. This woman, who was barely over 5'2" and looked so innocent, was a dominatrix who owned a dungeon and was teaching this muscled sex god how to use sex tools safely. A big grin lit up my face. I definitely wanted to participate in this late-night lesson. I asked if I could be an onlooker for the session and was grateful that they said yes. I'd never imagined I'd get the chance to see a dominatrix lesson at a sex dungeon. It seemed so impossible that I hadn't even put it on my bucket list.

It was my first time in a sex dungeon. Everything I'd seen in films, or my imagination, had misled me. We weren't in a basement with chains hanging from the wall, and a black-masked man didn't request a password. As we approached the unassuming building, my excitement grew. We walked up a flight of stairs in a residential building and into a studio apartment where we had to remove our shoes. Troy pulled back a curtain to reveal the main space. On the opposite side of the room was a cage on the floor big enough to fit a grown man and contraptions I couldn't identify. There was a bench that someone could lie on, with a cage underneath that a person could be locked in.

The class was now in session. Troy sat me down, handed me an excellent gin cocktail, and allowed me to observe. I watched in awe as this woman eagerly shared her knowledge with a man who was just as excited to learn how to please. They switched from dragon tail whips to leather paddles to combo floggers. Each tool had different techniques and rules so as not to hurt the person receiving the spanking. My mind was going a thousand miles a minute with curiosity and amusement. I asked questions along the way, and during their break, Troy began to show and explain her toy collection. I became a student in the world of kink and soaked up everything I could from this lesson.

The huge metal rig came with a backstory as it was custom-built. I let her know that I had never been suspended, because I felt as though I was too big to do it comfortably. In true dominant fashion, she said there was no such thing as being TOO BIG and all things could be done. For someone who battled insecurities with my body and weight, knowing that all things were possible despite the number on the scale made me excited about even more possibilities. I had felt too big in moments for a man to pick me up during sex. The fear of breaking something during the act or falling to the ground because I was too heavy often hindered me from openly exploring.

Next thing I knew, Troy was in between my legs, putting straps around each of my thighs, still in teacher mode. In a matter of minutes, my body was suspended in midair, quite securely, with both legs wide open, ready for a pounding. Well, not really. I was fully clothed the entire time, and the whole night was nothing more than witnessing a man's excitement about learning the proper ways to please a woman around her different touch points. There was a method to execute pain properly to be a mutually gratifying experience. This entire evening was so eye-opening. By this point in my life, I had quite a few friends who were sex workers, many of whom took pride in their careers. However, I'd never met people with this level of excitement around the art of pleasure.

I hadn't considered sex as something you worked to be better at before I got to my late twenties. Since I hadn't had proper sex education or people to talk about it with, I hadn't fully grasped how much I was responsible for and how I could find more enjoyment. Due to my insecurities, I'd normally let my partners take the lead and found most of my pleasure in doing what they wanted. Watching this level of attentiveness and study go into pleasure made me want to not only learn about ways I could please someone else, but also focus on my own needs.

It's important to find like-minded people on your journey of sex and self-discovery. Here are some things to ask yourself when doing an inventory check on the people around you.

- Does my inner circle allow me to express my sexual desires without shame?
- Do I feel like I can be my authentic self around the people I choose to hang with?
- Do my friends and potential partners align on the

same foundational core values when it comes to
navigating relationships?

- Can I learn to be a better person from my friends
  and community, and can they learn from me in
  turn?

- Have my friends created a safe space for me to
  express my concerns about my body, sex, and
  partners?

Now, these may seem like basic questions. However, if you sit down and apply these to your closest friends or lovers, you may be surprised to find some bad apples around you keeping you from being who you genuinely want and deserve to be. Many of us carry enough shame from the mistakes we've made and learned from to allow ourselves to be judged or ridiculed by those close by who remain ignorant. Once you make this assessment, you can choose to change your inner circle.

I was grateful to begin a friendship with Troy. We were definitely aligned. The next time I was invited to her dungeon, I would have another profound moment of insight. It was a weekend in New York when Black tech professionals from all over the country gathered for a conference. Troy had curated a night of sisterhood at her dungeon with eight Black women who found themselves in C-suite-level positions within their companies. They lived in places like Atlanta, Austin, and other cities within the tristate area. No, this wasn't a lesbian orgy taking place at a dungeon. Instead, in this space, we held room for one another to simply be. We discussed our hang-ups around dating and sex, how we navigated our roles in relationships outside of the patriarchal norm, and moments where we got to express our sexual desires with trustworthy partners. We giggled and gossiped over cocktails with cock rings in the background. There was comfort in sharing a room with strangers, with fellow women of color who felt safe enough to spill personal information about themselves.

Within the Black community, it can feel like people look the other way when it comes to discussing sex. The birds and the bees are often only discussed after it is too late. That is why this evening with Troy and these women was even more special. I didn't feel alone. I no longer felt like something was "wrong" with me and instead realized how unsafe and unsure many of us are about navigating the very thing that brought us into existence: sex. How had I never shared a space like this with other Black women, and why the fuck was it not happening more often?

When starting the podcast, our mission was to destigmatize sex within the Black community, specifically by having these conversations in a public setting. Variety, adventure, and taboo acts in the bedroom are often written off as "White People Shit," or what we call WPS. Due to centuries of trauma from slavery, American Black folks tend to shy away from conversations or activities that are overtly sexual in nature. Black bodies—especially Black women's bodies—were viewed as sex objects and often taken advantage of. BDSM and kink can raise concerns around the term "slave" and race play and whether it is appropriate for Black people to even engage in such behavior.

On our podcast, *WHOREible Decisions*, we spoke with porn star legends Nat Turnher and Mr. Marcus, as well as newcomer Jason Luv. The use of the N-word as a fetish came up in all three conversations. Non-Black men and women alike can have an itch to refer to Black men with the term that was rooted in hate for hundreds of years. There's an internal battle and ongoing conversation about the damaging treatment our ancestors endured and how it shows up for us today, even in the bedroom.

Kinky sex can also create misconceptions around identity. Sexual acts like cuckolding, pegging, rimming, submitting to a woman, or even moaning can incorrectly imply that Black men are less masculine. For Black women, acts are taboo when they are seen as unfeminine or unladylike—for example, having sex with more than one man at a time, exerting dominance over a man, spitting, swallowing, or engaging in anything beyond "regular" sex. To get to a healthy place where we can explore our sexuality, we must have conversations in accepting spaces and address the history of ourselves and our ancestors.

My third time at the dungeon was like a scene from one of those Zane books I grew up reading. I had been in a relationship with a man, who I was sure was my soulmate. We explored each other's bodies in ways I had never done before with a lover, and we pushed the boundaries to allow each other to experience every sexual inhibition. After an outing to a nude beach one weekend, I asked him if he'd like to join me at a sex dungeon. I told him my friend owned one and that we could use the dungeon for a night of excitement. Though I had been put into a rig and suspended during my first visit, I viewed Troy's place as a classroom. I had zero intention of going there to use any of the toys or engage in any actual penetration. However, during this next visit, the classroom would turn into my personal playroom.

It was a Saturday evening, so I figured this would be our warm-up before heading out to a sex club. He seemed excited and nervous, but I assured him that this was a comfortable space, and that Troy was a phenomenal host and teacher. We discussed the things we hadn't done yet but would consider trying on our drive over. We went back and forth and shared all of the random kinky memories we had of previous lovers, and it turned me on even more. Going to a dungeon was something new for him and something we would share together. I had never entered this space with a partner, so it felt almost surreal.

We walked in, and Troy greeted us with cocktails as we removed our shoes. She directed us into the main room and instructed us to sit in specific chairs. Though he could still see everything, he was in a seat of submission. Troy and I were seated in places of power and authority. She wanted him to know that she and I were equals and he was our sub. We sat for a while as he stared in awe at all of the sex toys that filled the walls and shelves. We had some casual conversation before things spiced up with his curiosity and questions about the contraptions. He loved to turn things into a game and said we should each pick something for the other to experience. I had mentioned before that I had never done electroplay and how I was a bit fearful of what the fuck electricity in the bedroom would even entail. I was adamant that it was some WPS. One of the devices that Troy had shown me before piqued my interest, and I knew immediately that I wanted to put his penis in a cage. The idea of locking up his dick turned me on. So, there it was: he would get to electrocute my pussy, and in return, I got to put his manhood into a chastity belt.

I smirked as I instructed my partner to take his pants off as Troy went to get the chastity belt. Troy gave me the silver metal contraption and began giving instructions on how to place his dick inside. It was more difficult than anticipated, so I needed help. In order to lock him in, he needed to be in soft gummy mode, but the feeling of four hands around his heavy dick made it grow. We tried so hard not to make this sensual, but what man could resist two women holding dick and balls in hand? We were fifteen minutes in with no success before I was given the job of making his dick soft again with conversation. I began talking politics as Troy continued to try to lock his penis up for me. With my help, we locked that penis on up. I sat looking at his naked body as cold metal entrapped the dick that was all mine. While he didn't seem to enjoy it much, it turned me on for him to trust me enough to have this experience with him. It was my turn next.

I was instructed to remove my clothes and lie on the bench in the center of the room underneath the rig. I propped up my legs as if a gynecologist were going to give me my annual pap smear. As I lay spread eagle, I got nervous; the idea of an electric current being enjoyable sounded almost like an oxymoron. I knew I enjoyed the stinging pain from a hand connecting with the softness of my ass and the pain from a large, throbbing dick opening up my pussy. But I could not imagine what enjoyable pain could come from electric currents.

Troy explained the tool that would be inserted in me: a clear glass cone with wires connected at the base operated by some control box. I was deadass about to allow a machine that looked like it was used to jump the dead battery of a car into my whole pussy. I was a big girl, though. He had allowed me to put him in such a vulnerable space, and I wanted him to be able to do the same. At the time, I thought less about the physical impact of this moment and leaned into the psychological. This allowed me and my partner to get closer. We were enjoying things for the first time together and removing fears because we trusted each other. Getting out of each of our comfort zones with each other provided us with an even stronger sexual bond.

The base of the tool was lubed and inserted into me. It was a bit cold, but it didn't feel any different from a glass dildo as it penetrated me. They began playing with the control, and I started to experience different waves vibrating the walls of my pussy. At first, my brain couldn't understand what was happening, so it took a while for me to relax and appreciate the sensation I was feeling. My partner asked if it hurt. In all seriousness, I almost couldn't find the words to describe what I felt. I told him it didn't hurt at all. They continued to press buttons on the motherboard, and that's when it happened. I had allowed myself to calm down enough to feel everything happening. I began to moan. My eyes rolled to the back of my head before I closed them. The only way I know how to describe this feeling is to say that it felt like eight tongues were inside of me at once, licking all of my walls. So many spots were being hit that I was convinced anatomically, we must have more than one G-spot, and so I don't know why these muthafuckas have such a hard time finding one. This immense feeling of pleasure actually scared me. I knew it was unrealistic to feel this every time, so I tried to compartmentalize the experience as it was happening. I moaned louder before I said, "Enough." I shared how fucking amazing this whole thing had felt and how I may have just experienced what it may be like to fuck an alien. But until they landed on this planet, I wasn't even going to get used to this incredible, out-of-this-world feeling inside my pussy.

While physically, this entire night was arousing in every way, the most memorable part of the evening was placing my vulnerability and trust in my partner while he did the same with me. We could talk about our fears, lusts, and desires and then act on them in a safe environment. This night brought us closer together. This night brought even more excitement to our relationship. This night was the seed that planted the root of our communication and allowed us to explore even more throughout our relationship. While finding out what you like and desire is essential, finding a partner to communicate and experience those things with may be just as important.

I want to share how difficult revisiting that last experience was when writing this chapter. I felt like I completely let a person all the way in that evening. When my ex and I broke up, it took months of therapy to be able to acknowledge the good moments the relationship provided for me. I hated him. He betrayed my trust in unimaginable ways. I felt like our entire relationship was built on lies. After all of his narcissistic, conniving behaviors, I struggled with feeling like anything over the three years was even real. I questioned if he ever loved me. I interrogated my own emotional and physical responses to him. I'm so proud to be in a space now where I can compartmentalize the moments of a failed relationship that served me and allowed me to grow. I am capable of trusting someone and letting them in. My walls can come down, and I have the capacity to love. While exploring my sexuality, it's been that much more rewarding and fun when I have found the right partner to do it all with.

I want to leave you with this because I hope that if you are interested in trying new things you will be open to talking to your partner about it.

INTRODUCING NEW IDEAS IN THE BEDROOM

COMMUNICATE, COMMUNICATE!—You cannot begin to introduce anything without talking to your partner first! For example, share porn of things you'd be interested in trying out and see their reaction. Use the video as your point of reference.

PLAN A FIELD TRIP TO THE SEX STORE—There are so many toys that many of us are unaware even exist. The sex store for adults is like the candy store for kids! It is a playground of wonders and can add to the excitement in the bedroom.

BE ACCEPTING OF YOUR PARTNER'S BOUNDARIES—Be OK with hearing "no" or "I don't think that's for me." You don't want to apply too much pressure about something your partner may not be interested in.

ADD "ADVENTURE" TO THE CALENDAR—Look forward to the spice! Put a date on the calendar when you will get kinky with it.

FEEL FREE TO TAKE THE LEAD—You can't expect your partner to read your mind! Be sure to advocate for your fantasies and desires. Buy the toy you want to try out! Try on a sexy negligee to boost your confidence in the bedroom.

Patriarchal Bullshit

"The Lord commands the wife to be submissive. Refusal to submit to the husband is therefore rebellion against God Himself. Submission to the husband is a test of her love for God as well as a test of love for her husband. The wife then must look upon her submission to her husband as an act of obedience to Christ and not merely to her husband."

—Wayne A. Mack (pastor and author of *Strengthening Your Marriage*)[1]

Matriarchal Reply

"The most 'emancipated' women . . . showed a far greater capacity for complete sexual enjoyment."

—Betty Friedan (activist and author of *The Feminine Mystique*)[2]

WHY STAND UP WHEN YOU CAN BE ON YOUR KNEES?

« WEEZY WTF »

TO START THIS chapter, I'd like to reference a 2018 *Vice* magazine article about the *WHOREible Decisions* podcast.

"The idea for *WHOREible Decisions* came to Weezy in 2016 when she was asked to guest star on the *No Chaser* podcast. 'I come into the recording session with a bag that had bondage tape, a collar, and a leash. I open it up, and they're looking at me like I'm crazy,' Weezy recalls to me inside the Downtown Manhattan studio where her and Mandii record *WHOREible Decisions*. 'The second we were done, they were like, "Yo, that was the most lit shit ever." When it came out, everybody loved it. They were getting crazy feedback. And I was like, *I need a podcast of my own, but who else do I know? Who's as much of a hoe as me?*"[3]

Mandii and I linked up, and the rest is history. To think that it all started with the spark of my sub energy.

Nate was the first guy from Tinder to whom I was hella pressed. At twenty-six, he hit all four of my requirements at the time.

1. FINE
2. TALL
3. BIG DICK
4. JOB

I didn't even really care about the job. I just needed to know that he could feed me. I used to always say on the podcast that I wanted the three Fs.

FUCK ME. FEED ME. FINANCE ME.

He was so much more than a simp, though. I met Nate for the first time around the corner from my house at a cute little bar on 54th Street. I never wanted to be far from my place, and traveling for dick I hadn't confirmed was good yet didn't make sense to me. My apartment at the time was a two-bedroom in Hell's Kitchen that my sugar daddy got me, but we'll dig into his old ass later.

When I walked into the bar, he was TOWERING over me. He was a cutie, 6'5", British accent, and boy-band hot. Okay, yes, he was a white guy, but the type that even Black girls want to fuck. Are you going to turn down Chris Hemsworth? No, bitch. No, you are not.

His first words were "Well, aren't you a little smoke show?" I was smiling from ear to ear! When I tell you he was undeniably sexy, he really was. Christian Grey had nothing on him (besides the private jet). He was so charismatic that it made it hard not to fall in love with him. He was completely aware of how attractive he was but still able to make you feel special, and that's a skill that a lot of good-looking people do not possess.

After a bunch of flirting and chatting about raving, drugs, and the New York City party scene, he stood up to use the restroom and kissed me before he walked away. That left me just enough time to send a mass group text about how I'd met my husband and would be living in London soon.

We ended the night around 11 p.m. and made plans to see each other again. Our next series of text messages was ALL about the sex—what the next time we see each other would be like, what I was into, what I wasn't. And then the real question: **Are you kinky?**

As someone who, at the time, knew that she liked spankings and had a threesome before . . . compared to other folks, YEAH, I WAS SUPER KINKY. Right?

He went on to tell me about how he was a Dom and asked me if I had ever been dominated. In my brain, that meant he was the aggressor, but that ain't the case for a REAL Dom. He had to do his checklist with me before I could submit. He'd already started the process by ensuring that our first get together was a vanilla meetup to get to know me in a safe setting, which can often be the first step in a Dom vetting a sub and vice versa. Next, he started to ask me questions so that he could get my pre-consent before engaging in impact play (what the fuck did that even mean?).

These questions aim to understand someone's BDSM preferences, practices, and community involvement. Here's an example of some of the things you may want to discuss with a prospective partner:

LIMITS: Hard limits are activities they absolutely won't engage in. Soft limits are activities they are hesitant about but might consider under certain circumstances.
FORMS OF BDSM: Types of BDSM practices they enjoy or seek in a relationship (e.g., bondage, dominance/submission, sadomasochism).

PARTNER PREFERENCES: Whether they prefer a single partner or are open to multiple partners in their BDSM activities.

REAL LIFE VS. ONLINE: If they engage in BDSM practices in person, online, or both.

COMMUNITY INVOLVEMENT: Their level of activity in the local BDSM community, such as attending events, munches, or being part of BDSM groups. (A munch is a casual social gathering for people involved in or interested in kink, BDSM alternative relationship lifestyles, or fetishes. No BDSM, kink, or fetish activities take place, however.)

VIEWS ON SAFEWORDS: Asking what their safeword is to ensure safety and consent during BDSM activities.

SADISM AND MASOCHISM: Whether they identify as a sadist (someone who enjoys inflicting pain) or a masochist (someone who enjoys receiving pain) and to what extent.

PROTOCOLS: Specific behaviors or rituals they expect from themselves or their partner(s) within a BDSM context.

PUNISHMENTS: Examples of punishments they might use or expect as part of their BDSM dynamics (e.g., spanking, corner time, verbal reprimands).

These questions can help build an understanding of an individual's BDSM preferences and boundaries.

I've learned that I am a masochistic submissive. Submission could be thought of as weak because the word means "the action or fact of accepting or yielding to a superior force or to the will or authority of another person."[4] But to be a sexual sub, you actually have to be mentally strong. Submission is NOT for the weak. I know for a fact how much power I possess when I'm a sub. Many people couldn't handle the level of pain or domination I've experienced. In genuine consensual BDSM, the sub IS the master. We ask for what we want. We are the key holders to the sick, dirty, nasty pleasure that we're seeking! The submissive has a significant say in what will and won't happen, and this negotiation process demonstrates our power. The sub often influences the emotional and psychological aspects of the relationship. Our reactions, responses, and emotional state can guide the Dominant's actions and decisions, creating a balanced dynamic where both parties' well-being is prioritized. Most important of all, you've got to realize that, like any other relationship, a healthy BDSM relationship is built on mutual respect. The Dominant respects the submissive's limits, boundaries, and autonomy, acknowledging that the submissive's participation is a gift, not a right.

Nate was a kinky motherfucker. He brought up sexual things I had never imagined. He shared a photo of a girl with a stocking over her face and his cum all over it. He told me all about his kinks and what he'd like to watch me do, like double penetration with him and another guy. Nate was my entrance into an entirely new world. I had done my Black girl's due diligence. I read Zane and Eric Jerome Dickey, and I watched all the best porn stars in action. *Fifty Shades of Grey* had come out a few years before meeting him, but it wasn't necessarily the real lives people were living. WAS IT?

Nate was the REAL deal. The first time we slept together, I feel like Nate would say it was vanilla. It was after our third date (my usual rule). He came back to my place, and I remember seeing his face when he got upstairs.

"WHAT THE FUCK?"

That's how impressive my place was at The Marc—forty-four floors up, floor-to-ceiling windows, and a second bedroom just for my clothes. I remember him joking about whether I was a secret drug dealer or not, and typically, I would have lied about how I'd got this apartment. But Nate had shared everything with me, even photos of women with stockings over their faces looking like kidnapping victims. Why not be honest with him? I told him all about my sugar daddy back in Orlando.

This kinky muthafucka turned my sugar daddy into a whole-ass role play.

We sat on my couch, and I expected the shame to roll in when he said, "So, you enjoy being paid, don't you?"

I didn't even realize what this was turning into until we were rolling around in the bedroom full of furniture my SD had purchased: my California king with Egyptian cotton sheets, the white chaise against the window overlooking the Hearst Tower, and the full-length mirror shipped in from Italy that we watched ourselves in like a movie.

I remember this being an exhilarating moment and secretly praying he would stay over. I wasn't used to men getting up and leaving, but Nate was definitely a "respectful" fuck buddy. We probably got thirty minutes into whatever bullshit I'd thrown on the TV before his cuddles turned into an arm stretch and, "All right, guess I'll be heading back to Brooklyn now." It was all good, though. I needed space from him to start planning our future kids' names.

Seriously, though, he may have been one of the most handsome men I'd ever seen. Low-key, if he weren't white, he would have been the type I wanted to marry, but in reality, Trump had just become president (for the first time), and shit was getting too dicey.

Regardless, we didn't have a deep connection. He was just a sucker for my big bright eyes when he talked about his world and his eagerness to show it to me.

A day or two after our first encounter, he sent a follow-up text about how amazing that night was and how he was getting hard thinking about me. A sexy pic of me was required, of course; I ran to the bathroom at work to send the requested photo of my boobs, but no. In true Dom fashion, Nate wanted to give me my orders. He wanted me to find a place in the office to take it and sneak the photo while my colleagues weren't looking.

I think I even had a time limit, and when I wasn't moving fast enough, he let me know how much I was fucking boring him. NOT MY FUTURE HUSBAND, but A GOOD DOM.

I rushed to a conference room, snapped a pic, and finally got the text that every sub desires:

"Good Girl."

I mean it when I tell you I had no prior BDSM experience before this relationship. Every sub and Dom must be born with this shit, though. How did I know exactly what to do? How to respond? The voice to use? Had I been practicing and didn't even know it? Nate gave me the safe space and guidance to learn how to ask for what I wanted.

Most of our discovery happened as we texted. We both had day jobs that we were bored at, so what better time to text about punishments than on the clock? Nate would send me links and photos to check my temperature and what I could be down for—things like restraints, bound ankles and wrists, and sometimes even just the language surrounding certain sex acts. I realized I never really liked the word "bitch." I require my derogatory statements wrapped up in a lil' bow or something.

"Good little slut."

"MY perfect slut."

I loved the possession surrounding some of the BDSM language. MINE. OWN. Giving myself up to someone is truly my biggest kink in life, and Nate taught me that.

The second time he was inside me was in the middle of the day. After a few more text exchanges, he checked in with me about trust and safety. Nate asked me if I would allow him to take control of me. Of course, I said YES. Not that I knew what it meant. The only rules I had at the time were to pick my safeword and be waiting in my apartment with lingerie. I was nervous for the twenty-four hours leading up to seeing him and planned my excuse to leave work early. I had to do my routine! I told my boss I had to scout a company uptown, made a fake calendar invite, and headed back to my apartment. I ran myself a bath, did a full-body scrub, exfoliated, and did that shave where your foot is on the wall so you can make sure to get every microscopic hair.

I was on the couch watching *Sex and the City* to distract myself when I got a text message with more orders. He told me that I was to be waiting in my foyer with my back to the door, sitting up straight on the floor with my hands on my knees. I was only to speak when spoken to. I had a time range of about an hour for his arrival and had to be on the floor the entire time. My doorman was given his name before he got there so I wouldn't have to get up and answer the phone.

My pussy was so fucking wet. I remember squealing a few times in excitement and feeling silly because I was all alone in my apartment. I had secretly asked my doorman to ping me once he was on the elevator so I could look like perfection before Nate walked in the door. I wanted him to see the arch in my back and my tiny little waist CLEARLY.

He put his things down, told me how sexy I looked, told me to choose a safeword, and proceeded to put a blindfold over my eyes.

I was terrified and excited. I tried not to smile so that I didn't appear to be as inexperienced as I was, but fuck was this shit exhilarating! I couldn't see anything; it was pitch black on a bright summer day. I listened intently for Nate's next instruction.

He told me to be still, keep my blindfold on, and hold my hands behind my back.

Since I couldn't see him, I followed the sounds of his footsteps as he walked around my apartment. He fixed himself a drink at my bar; I could hear him pouring and sipping, then putting the rocks glass down on the table next to me.

I was still on my knees at the doorway, pussy DRIPPING!

I remember precisely how horny I was that day. I'd seen the white in my panties, so I knew I was ovulating. I always find it so sexy to tell someone how creamy I am, but fuck it, he'd find out soon enough.

Nate stood in front of me. I could smell him as he approached. I heard his belt buckle unlatch, the zip as he pulled his zipper down, and his jeans dropping to the floor.

"Open your mouth."

I started to laugh because, frankly, how the hell was I supposed to find his dick if I couldn't see it or grab it?

He asked, "What's so funny?"

I said, "I'm sorry, sir. It's just that I feel silly because I don't know where it is."

His voice became deeper and sterner when he said, "Well, open your mouth and find it."

I craned my neck and stuck out my tongue, trying to go in the right direction, and finally, I could taste him. He was a mix of that sweet and salty taste. It's like a little bit of man sweat but just enough musk to turn you on. I had my entire mouth around his dick, and I was worried about going for my usual slow licks because I didn't want to lose it.

I started forcing myself down his dick so I could choke and have a mouth full of that thick mucus spit. Since he was so big, it was easy. He grabbed the back of my head so as not to move the blindfold and started face fucking me. It was so HOT!

I was scared my neighbors would hear me. My apartment was close to the elevator, and we were still by the front door where he'd told me to wait. I shifted my body to spread my knees a bit more so that I could put my pussy closer to the floor just to have some friction.

Fuck, I was so horny, and I couldn't even touch myself since my hands were ordered to be behind my back.

I raised my hand to ask a question in the middle of giving him head.

"WHAT?" He groaned.

"Can I please touch my pussy, sir?"

He gave me a little light slap on the face and said, "You can't do ANYTHING unless I tell you to."

(I think I love him.)

After my chest was soaked with spit and precum, he told me to remove my hands from behind my back and crawl, following the sound of his voice.

Thank goodness! I needed a little stretch. I got down on all fours, arched my back, and crawled toward him. He didn't even need to speak. I could FEEL his heat.

He gave me all the affirmation I needed, telling me how sexy I was, what a perfect little slut I was for him, and how impressed he was with me.

He used his arms to lift me onto my couch and told me I deserved a reward.

He slid off my panties, let them hang around one of my ankles, and started licking me from my toes all the way to the edge of my vulva. Breathing all over my pussy, but not swallowing me whole. It drove me CRAZY! He was such a good tease.

He stuck his finger deep inside me, and when he pulled it out, I could hear the sound of him sucking the juices off. "Damn, you taste so amazing."

I was moaning in delight, and I wasn't even being stimulated. I asked him, "When can I see you?"

He said, "Not until I'm inside of you."

He stood over me, making sure to drag his dick along my face so that I knew to open my mouth for him again. I was laid down on the couch, my head dangling over the sectional so he could adequately throat fuck me. Slightly dizzy but staying in the game, I gave him the sloppiest head to ensure he would never stop coming back to me. There was so much spit spilling all over my face it began to get stuck in my lashes and my nose, but I didn't care! Getting face fucked is an ultimate sexual act to me. Although gross, the feeling of almost throwing up and having to control my gag reflex gets me hot, and sometimes I want it to the point that my eyes are fucking bulging. A nice messy little bitch with smeared makeup, out of breath from the choking, and a little slap in the middle of it are the rewards I like to receive.

When I'm in complete submission, I am so ready to serve that there isn't an inconvenience that would keep me from making him cum. Finally, it got to the point where it was unbearable. He picked me up, cleaned me off with whatever was nearby, and went to get a condom. While he was ripping it open, I had my fingers in between my legs, making sure I was as wet as he needed me to be so that he could enter me as promised. I felt him fill me up before he suddenly ripped the mask off.

"Hi," he said when he smiled at me.

He gave me a lovely kiss, told me how much of a good girl I had been, and stroked me while he kept a hand on my neck. Using me as his anchor, he was careful not to choke me too hard—just enough so that I got a little red in the face. After fifteen minutes of mind-blowing sex (of course, no more than that; he was about to explode from all that foreplay), he laid me down on the leather chaise that my sugar daddy had bought for my apartment and told me to stick my tongue out.

I stayed reclined while he jerked the cum out of his dick, using me as a visual, while I kept a finger on my clit to make sure I was gettin' mine, too. My eyes were closed when I felt the warm splatter of his cum all over my face. I opened them back up once the coast was clear and watched him squeeze the remaining semen out of the tip of his dick. I licked it up like an ice cream cone as he fed the rest to me during cleanup.

He pulled me onto the bed and cuddled me for a while, telling me how sexy it was and thanking me for allowing him to play out that particular scene. We talked more about our boundaries and things we would like to try next.

Nate was an amazing example of confident, consensual, and cocky. He was badass enough to lead us into a scene that felt real, cautious enough to make sure I was comfortable, and arrogant enough to make me feel like he was the ONLY man who could be my Dom.

Many people proclaim that they're Doms just because they like "rough sex," but without safe and consensual awareness, rough sex practices can lead to injuries or even death.

Asphyxiation or choking, for example, can seem like such a "basic" form of BDSM, but there are a few tips I'd implore you to practice before engaging.

- **CHOOSE A SAFE GESTURE**—Choking can leave you
  literally speechless and unable to use a safeword; my
  preferred safe gesture is a "tap out."
- **KEEP YOUR HANDS ON THE DOM'S WRISTS**—I like
  to squeeze when I'm ready for more choking, and it
  also eases my brain knowing my hands are on top of
  my Dom's so that I have a feeling of control or that
  I'm able to pull away.

To this day, this experience with Nate remains in my top three
sex moments of all time. I'm so grateful I took a chance on spon-
taneity and allowed myself to experience the type of pleasure I had
only read about in silly erotica books or watched in porn.

If this story has made you a little curious about exploring your
submissive side, here are a few key items you MUST have in your
nightstand.

- **A BALL GAG**—All subs need to know how to shut
  the fuck up!
- **SOME FORM OF RESTRAINT/BONDAGE**—Most like
  handcuffs, but I prefer sex tape—it's tape you can
  buy at an adult store that binds to itself and not
  your skin.
- **A LEASH**—I have a dog, so this part came cheap, but
  you get the drift.

Asking for someone to dominate you is no walk in the park.
Luckily, Nate was an expert, but I still knew I deeply desired to be
a sub.

Here are three questions to ask yourself before engaging in submission:

1. Is this MY choice without the pressure of my partner wanting to be dominant or tame me?
2. Do I truly feel power by *asking* for this?
3. Do I believe that I am capable of experiencing pleasure through pain and/or humiliation?

If you answered YES to all three, get ready to be a good little girl or boy!!!

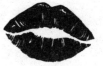

Patriarchal Bullshit
"Everything in woman is a riddle, and everything in woman hath one solution—it is called pregnancy."
—Friedrich Nietzsche (philosopher, scholar, and author of *Thus Spoke Zarathustra*)[1]

Matriarchal Reply
"I have built an incredible life. I have become a woman that I am proud to be. And then someone tells me about their friend who adopted a child at 52 and how 'it's never too late for your life to have meaning,' and my worth gets diminished as I am reminded that I have 'failed' on the marriage and carriage counts. Me! This bold, liberated, independent woman."
—Tracee Ellis Ross (actress and *Glamour*'s 2017 Women of the Year Summit speaker)[2]

WHY DON'T THEY JUST CALL IT A VACUUM?*

« MANDII B »

THEY SAY THAT women always know when something is off in their bodies, as if we have a magical, intuitive gift. In my case, this didn't feel like a gift. It felt like a damn curse. I suspected what was going on before the test gave me a concrete answer. It was just a gut feeling, but I knew the inevitable had happened. Maybe it is a form of innate programming meant to ensure that the species will survive. Was I supposed to feel some attachment and go into a protective mode where I would take better care of myself and, therefore, be part of the chain of life, ensuring that there would be one more human in the world? If so, my programming must have been way off; the protective and nurturing feeling never kicked in. Some women might feel guilty that they don't feel an immediate sense of maternal instinct, but I'm not one of them. And though the idea that we are all meant to be mothers is slowly changing in the "rich auntie" era, there are a lot of people who still believe in that antiquated notion.

I think this "maternal lie" was created and perpetuated by men, who will never understand what it is to carry a life inside of them. This must be the case because 625,978 abortions for 2021 were reported to the CDC from 48 reporting areas in the United States.[3] Remember that these are just those that were reported, because we damn well know that not all of them were. In 2021, the abortion rate was 11.6 abortions per 1,000 women aged 15–44 years, and the abortion ratio was 204 abortions per 1,000 live births.[4] Sadly, I understand that some of these women wanted to carry their pregnancies to term and were unable to because of extenuating circumstances. But there were also a lot of women who chose to have an abortion for various personal reasons. How many of your friends and relatives have had abortions? Personally, I can say that the list of people I know who've had abortions is longer than those who haven't.

I'm sharing my story with you at a time when we are going through what feels like a horrifying dystopian shift here in the United States when it comes to women's rights. Well, at least if you're liberal. *The Handmaid's Tale* seems like a possible reality and that has me shook! Like so many others, I never thought I would live to see the day *Roe v. Wade* was overturned. But in June 2022, the U.S. Supreme Court, run by a conservative majority, did just that and opened the door for states to ban abortion outright. In the years since the ruling, fourteen states have made abortion illegal. That means that nearly 22 million women (in addition to people who may not identify as women but are capable of becoming pregnant) of reproductive age—almost one in three—found themselves living in states where abortion is unavailable or severely restricted. Before *Roe v. Wade* was overturned, getting an abortion was already difficult for many people—especially those who faced steep barriers to accessing health care, including people with low incomes, Black and Brown people, immigrants, young people, people with disabilities, and people in rural populations. This prejudice is likely to worsen as clinic-based abortion care disappears in many states, several of them clustered in regions like the South.

When I found myself in need of an abortion, I was living in Atlanta, and I was facing a couple of the barriers that I just mentioned. I was a sixteen-year-old poverty-stricken Brown girl. But something felt off, so I decided to figure out if my instincts were correct even though I hadn't missed my period yet. I was on a mission to get an answer, and I knew what I had to do. I got dressed and took the short walk to the Kroger grocery store on Chamblee Tucker Road, where I found the pregnancy tests. I wasn't thrilled when I saw they were behind one of those plastic lockboxes, and I had to find someone to get one for me. Since COVID-19, they've locked up damn near everything, depending on what neighborhood you live in. But back then, it felt to me like they locked up the things associated with sex and contraception—you know, the things that we were supposed to be ashamed of. We needed a store clerk for everything from the Plan B pill to pregnancy tests and even condoms sometimes. Here I was with a stranger all in my business. But I thought, *Fuck it, let me buy this test and get this shit over with.* I have always been smart enough to know that knowledge is power. With the answers, I can make my decisions clearly and ascertain my next move.

After paying for the test and grabbing a Gatorade just in case I had trouble peeing, I went directly into the bathroom at the store. Luckily, it turned out to be a single-stall restroom, so I had some privacy and time to myself. I read the directions, tore open the box, and unwrapped the stick. I made sure to follow the instructions and "point the absorbent tip downward into your urine stream." While doing this, I also pissed on my hand more than I pissed on the damn stick. Then I put the cap back on and laid the stick on the corner of the sink, washed my hands, and waited out my three minutes, which felt like a million years. You know how you conveniently remember to talk to God when you're in trouble? Well, that's what I started to do. I began a dialogue with God or someone, and then I convinced myself that I'd hyped myself up for no reason at all, that I had myself worked up like I always did before a big school test. My fears were always unfounded, and I would always ace the test. And then I looked down and realized that I had aced this test, too, because the second faint pink line had appeared.

I was not willing to believe that this was true. I reread the directions on the box; I took the second test and looked at the expiration dates. I had decided that everything else was to blame, and the world had turned upside down, because there was no way in hell that I was pregnant!

I didn't think this could happen in my first year of having sex. Somehow, I figured that you'd have to be having sex for years before you could actually get pregnant. I was an overachiever; I got straight A's, played all the sports, worked and paid my own way, and had a car. This didn't happen to girls like me; this happened to other girls. When the second test was also positive, I had to take a deep breath and be completely honest with myself—I knew exactly how this had happened. That summer was the first time my sister and I had been sent to stay with my dad in Florida. While I was there, I'd had unprotected sex with a guy they called Elmo. And I am pretty sure that no one in life has ever hoped to get knocked up by someone who was given their nickname because (a) Elmo the Muppet is red, and (b) they happened to be a member of the gang

Bloods. And I hate to drag Weezy's ass into this, but that bitch was the reason I had met Elmo in the first place—not to be confused with placing blame on her for my poor decisions.

My dad only knew that I was staying at my friend Weezy's house with her and her parents. As you know by now, they were rich as hell, so I'm sure he assumed I was safe there. He had no way of knowing that we were running all over the place and doing whatever we wanted. At the time, Weezy had a crush on this rapper she'd met on MySpace, and he had invited her to go to his show in Tampa. The rapper promised to get us a hotel room if we got ourselves there. I was excited. I was like, "Bitch, let's go." We hopped on an Amtrak from Orlando to Tampa. It was only an hour or so ride, and when we got to the hotel, it turned out to be a motel. It looked like The Dunes from *Insecure*, and yes, I know those are apartments, but you get the picture. We didn't care; we were sixteen and had our own room! When the rapper showed up with his friends, beer, and Smirnoff, we were ready to party. Elmo was this skinny guy who wandered in with dreads and brought the drugs. Weezy and I didn't do that kind of shit at the time, but we definitely drank.

We all hung out and chilled for a while, and then everyone started to leave, and Weezy and her guy also went out. When they left, Elmo and I started making out, and clearly, we ended up doin' the damn thing. From what I remember, the sex was great, or however "great" sex really is when you're young and inexperienced. We went several rounds, and at first, we started off using a condom, but after a couple of rounds, my head was in the clouds. He promised that he would pull out. That good ol' having faith in a man pulling out has gotten a lot of us, huh? I was still tipsy, and I'm not even sure if I was paying attention to whether he did. He and I kept fucking and talking all night long. But the next day, Weezy and I had to hop on the Amtrak and head back to Orlando. Elmo put his phone number into my pink champagne–colored Motorola Razr phone, and I told him I lived in Atlanta. I told him he should fly out to see me, and I thought that was that.

My sister and I left Florida the weekend of the Fourth of July and went back home to be with my mom. Elmo and I texted and talked on the phone a lot. I was surprised to feel like I was vibing with him and genuinely liked him. I found out that he had a three-year-old daughter already. That didn't bother me because, at this time, many of the boys at my school had begun having kids. Before I took the test, I'd asked him how many times he thought he'd cum with me. He counted five or six. So, to be fair, I literally knew how I'd gotten there. This made me even more nervous, because, in my mind, that number hadn't exceeded three. I put the tests into my pocket and walked home. My head was spinning, and I was trying to figure out how I was going to tell my mom. But I want you to understand that I had already made my decision. I knew what I wanted to do. I was not ready to be a mom!

I knew what I wanted, but Planned Parenthood says that you have the following choices:

PARENTING: Giving birth and raising the child.
ABORTION: Ending the pregnancy.
ADOPTION: Giving birth and placing the child with another person or family forever.

Finding out you're pregnant can feel overwhelming, but try to stay calm. You're going to be okay, and there are people who can help you. You can find a link to Planned Parenthood for more information at the end of this chapter.

My mom was working overnight, so when I got back to our place, she was in her room asleep. She had these heavy blackout curtains so that she could sleep during the day. I was crying, and when I opened the door, I began crying even harder. I flicked on the light, slowly approached her bed, and watched her look at me with confusion. I then flung the pregnancy sticks on her bed and screamed through my tears, "I don't want it!" My mom, now wide awake, stared at me in disbelief before tears filled her eyes. She said that she needed a minute to process what the hell was going on, and I immediately felt like I had let her down. Not that we ever talked about the birds and the bees, but I just knew my mom didn't expect this to be a reality for me at my age. I went to my room and waited for her.

While working on this chapter, I had a discussion with my mom about what she remembered. This was the first time we had talked about my abortion in seventeen years. Isn't that interesting? So many of us have been through this, yet we are given few forums to discuss it openly. Or maybe we carry shame and don't want to reopen this wound we now live with. Abortion is something that my mom had experienced, too, but in her story, she wasn't given a choice. She was told what her decision would be. Because of that, when my mom came to my room to talk to me, she made it clear that she wanted me to think about my decision. This was the first time she shared her experience with abortion with me. She'd had her first abortion because she was forced into it by her super racist stepfather. After all, the father of the baby was Black. At the time, she wanted to keep her baby. She knew at an early age that she wanted to be a mother. When her stepfather told her she wouldn't be, he followed up by making my mom call the father of the child and said, "Tell that nigger you killed his baby." My heart dropped hearing this. This explained why I had probably only seen my step-grandfather twice and didn't know much about my mom's side of the family. So, when it came to making my choice, she wanted to ensure that I knew she would support me either way.

But I was super clear on my decision: I had a vision of what I wanted my life to be and everything I wanted to achieve. I had too many things to do; at this time in my life, I envisioned myself attending Duke University and playing basketball on a scholarship. I didn't even have a passport yet, but I knew I wanted to travel the world and possibly study abroad. I was clear about the fact that a baby was not a part of this picture.

My mom says she wishes she'd had this conversation with me earlier and that it wasn't in the form of a trauma bond. No one had talked to her, either, so this was part of our familial cycle. She said she would have talked to me earlier about the consequences and results of the actual "birds and bees," but here is the issue: the problem is a cyclical one. Before she got pregnant at fifteen, no one had ever talked to her about sex, either. Though we're from different generations, my mom and I both remember being told very little at school. She didn't have Planned Parenthood or any resources at the time in New Port Richey, Florida, where she grew up. I remember a sex ed class where we—and when I say *we*, I mean the young women—were told by our teacher to abstain from having sex. The boys were going to be boys, and the girls were going to stay angelic virgins somehow. Math is my strong suit, and I remember thinking about how it would work in real time. That math was not mathing. We were told not to have sex because we would either (a) get pregnant, (b) get HIV or some other sexually transmitted disease that would make you filthy, or (c) all the above. Welp! I was battling the multiple-choice selection here, being (a).

The next day, after doing some research, my mom told me that the abortion would cost around five hundred dollars. We immediately tried to figure out where that money would come from. Mom worked sixty hours a week and, even with her overtime, made just enough to cover the bills. When we returned from being with Daddy, she had just surprised my sisters and me with new bedroom sets, so her funds were depleted. So, I did the next logical thing and called up Elmo; I knew he had the money to help because he was dealing. When he picked up the phone, I told him my feeling had been correct, but I also told him not to worry because I wasn't keeping it. His immediate response was insane; this fucker had the nerve to say to me that he wouldn't give me the money because he wasn't going to let me kill his son. His son? Now this man was a prophet who already knew the sex of the baby? I obviously couldn't count on him, and all the feelings I thought I'd had dissipated immediately. After I told my mom what Elmo had said, she told me I would have to ask Daddy. Dad always had money, so he could've helped. I felt a pit in my stomach at having to call my dad and tell him the news. In his heavy Jamaican accent, his reply was "That's not my problem. Ya'll figure it out." Maybe it was ego, and this happening while I was in his care made him feel like a failure as a father, but this became one of the many reasons a strain has remained in our relationship. No one else in our family had the cash to help us; a couple hundred dollars would set any of them back.

My mom came up with one hundred dollars, and I had some money saved from my summer in Florida, but we still needed about three hundred dollars. Since this was a time-sensitive matter, I racked my brain to think of anyone who could help me. Allie was my close friend. Through our relationship, I was introduced to her new friend Keda. Now, I didn't have anything against this girl, but she wasn't exactly my favorite person because, in my mind, she'd stolen my friend. I texted Keda and asked if we could talk, but she happened to be at work (the fact that she had a job was why she was the only person I could think of asking). Keda texted back and said she was on her break at Coldstone, so I could call her.

I was nervous about talking to Keda because we were not very close, and we had hung out a few times and shared a few three-way calls. We were only ever together when we were with Allie. I tried to make small talk for the first couple minutes before I finally told her what was happening. It took everything in me, but finally, I asked if she could lend me the money to assist with the cost of my very big mistake. To give you some context, Keda's dad had died the year before, so she was working because she had to. She helped support the household financially in the absence of the man of the house. She was working to survive, but didn't hesitate to say, "Yes, I'll help you. I can lend you the money." She said she knew then that if I had asked her of all people, I needed it more than she did. For me to ask her when we were not that tight, she knew that I was desperate. I told her I would pay her back in two weeks, and she sent me the money via a Western Union wire. This was before the days of Venmo, Cash App, and Zelle. With the funds in place, my mom made my appointment and took a night or two off of work to be sure to have time with me after the procedure.

The clinic wasn't like anything I'd seen on the news or TV. There were no protestors outside. I didn't have to walk through a crowd of people calling me a murderer. It was quiet, and when we got inside, the mood was somber. My mom and I were struck by all the different types of people in the waiting room. There were other young girls like me and women well into adulthood. Some women sat with friends for support. The young girls appeared to all be accompanied by their moms or mother figures. Some of the ladies were even supported by their romantic partners. They called me to the back, and my mom sat nervously, waiting for me, as she wasn't allowed to join me. She says that she felt sad but knew she had helped me make the right decision for me at the time.

When I got to the back, they did a sonogram and showed me a picture of the baby. They wanted to be sure that I wanted to go through with it. I don't remember having any attachment to the dot I saw on the paper. It honestly made me feel even more disconnected; it was the size of a ballpoint pen tip, and it didn't have any attributes that would make me think, *Oh, look, there is my child.* Now, this may sound heartless, but there was not an arm, not a leg, not a head, not a foot—nothing. When they insisted that I was six weeks along, I knew that I was four weeks and two days along, so I accused them of lying to me. I didn't trust these people and told them I knew what I wanted to do. They spent more time than I would have liked trying to convince me that I shouldn't be making this decision. I lay down on the table in my dressing gown and told myself I was doing the right thing. And then I heard the sound of the machine they used, and the hum sounded just like a vacuum. Being the black-and-white thinker that I am, I knew that, realistically, that was what was happening.

They were sucking this dot out of my womb.

I went home, and when I tried to let Elmo know it was done, I found out he had gotten locked up. I took this as a further sign that I had made the right choice. Even so, I couldn't eat anything that night. The next day, I still didn't have any appetite. My mind was all over the place. My mom took me to Arby's and gave me a pill that she told me would help me to eat. I took that pill and decimated a roast beef and cheddar sandwich, my first meal in thirty-six hours. My mom sat back, watching me, and said, "Girl, that wasn't any pill to make you eat! I just gave your ass Tylenol." My mom knew that my not eating had more to do with my psychological state. At that point, I didn't care because it worked. I went back to school the following week. I had missed the first week of school and cared more about missing the first week of training for the volleyball season than the fact I had just experienced an abortion. No one there ever knew what had happened. The only thing I had left to do was pay back Keda—because I don't like owing anyone. Although it took me six weeks to wire the money back and not two, after I paid her back, she and I never spoke about it again, until I started working on this section of the book.

Writing this chapter has made me go back and speak to the women in my life who were there for me during that time. I know that sharing this story is essential. I had pushed this experience to the back of my mind for all these years. As demonstrated by my lack of appetite, I inherently felt some guilt after the experience. Or maybe it was the shame of letting myself down. I didn't know that I was doing what was right for me because of some preconditioned notion that I had done something "wrong" in the eyes of society. The fact that it took me writing this to make me have an open dialogue about abortion is part of the issue. If we stay silent, we feel separate from one another, which is a huge part of the problem. We are not separate; abortion is something that many of us or the people that we love have experienced. If we don't start speaking up about our experience with choosing not to keep a baby as a necessary option, those with conservative views will have an easier time controlling our narratives.

I have also come to realize that this experience may have led to my advocacy about contraception and protected sex as an adult. I absolutely LOVE condom sex and have zero desire to have sex casually without protection. I find it mind-boggling how using condoms is no longer the norm despite more people engaging in frivolous sex. Raw sex does not make a man like you more, nor does it mean your connection to him is any closer than if you use a condom.

We have to continue to fight for our right to make choices about our bodies without shame. I'm not trying to say that I have the answers to an issue that we have been trying to figure out for decades. I am saying that when my time came, I was grateful that I could make a choice. I feel every woman, no matter the circumstances, should also be able to make her own decision.

ABORTION INFORMATION & RESOURCES

- PLANNED PARENTHOOD—PlannedParenthood.org /learn/abortion
- CENTER FOR REPRODUCTIVE RIGHTS— ReproductiveRights.org
- NATIONAL ABORTION FEDERATION—ProChoice.org
- REPRODUCTIVE FREEDOM FOR ALL— ReproductiveFreedomForAll.org/resources /resources-for-accessing-abortion-care/
- HEY JANE—HeyJane.com/resources

Patriarchal Bullshit

"When a strong woman recklessly throws away
her strength she is worse than a weak woman
who has never had any strength to throw away."
—Thomas Hardy (poet and author of
Far from the Madding Crowd)[1]

Matriarchal Reply

"You think he belongs to you because you want
to belong to him. . . . Don't. It's a bad word, 'belong.' Especially when you put it with somebody you love.
Love shouldn't be like that."
—Toni Morrison (author of *Song of Solomon* and
the first African American woman to win
the Nobel Prize in Literature in 1993)[2]

WHEN DO YOU KNOW YOU'VE STAYED TOO LONG?

« WEEZYWTF »

I HADN'T REALLY considered that the high highs only exist if we also know the feeling of the lowest of lows. Life is a series of contrasts, and the longer that I'm here, the more I can recognize this fact.

I never realized until recently that the way men had treated and cheated on me had patterns that have contributed to my overall sex life. The worst part about some of what's happened as part of my cycle of trauma and PTSD is that I've engaged in sexual acts that I would normally have taken pleasure in, but would have been safer and healthier with another person.

After my breakup with Scissors, I went on to meet Ol Bae, a Brooklyn native who was handsome, refined, successful, and perfect on paper. I met him at an exclusive industry event held at an upscale bowling alley in Midtown. Mandii and I had both been invited as the podcast was growing in popularity.

I saw him the second I walked in. He had this big smile and was so fucking confident. He was only 5'11", but he walked around like he was ten feet tall. The first time he approached me at the party was because a woman I was next to started flirting with him. This lady is a well-known personality who's even been on our show, but sadly, I can't spill that tea. She asked him if he wanted to join her later for drinks, and he replied, "Only if she comes," his finger pointed at me. I said something to brush him off since my associate had an interest in him, and walked away. But I did feel that thing when you just know . . . this man is going to be a part of my story for better, worse, or that more realistic combination of both.

After another hour, he scurried up to me with a rush of frenetic energy.

Ol Bae: Hurry up and give me your number. I'm about to leave.
Me: Ummmm . . . For what?
Ol Bae: Ha! What the fuck you mean, for what? I don't need a reason. Give it to me because I want it.
Me: If you don't give me a reason, then I won't give you my number.
Ol Bae: Fine. Because you're pretty and because I know you feelin' me like I am feelin' you.

He wasn't wrong . . .

Ol Bae: Hurry up and put your digits in my phone.

And I did.

Ol Bae: My car is already downstairs.

I remember thinkin' I had just met the most Brooklyn nigga ever. And I also knew I was looking good that night. He texted me his name and told me to lock him in before I'd even left the party. Of course, I didn't respond until a day later. Gotta keep it playa!

A week or so later, I met him at a speakeasy in Chinatown. He was twenty minutes late and seemed disinterested in anything that I had to say, which was a disappointment considering how eager he had been to get to know me more just a few nights before.

I listened to HIM talk about his amazing life, all the places he traveled to, the connections he had, the designer shows he'd been to—a life that I felt I was on the cusp of. Or, at least, wanted to be. When I talked about myself, he was detached, his eyes darting around the room. Finally, bored by me, he interrupted me and asked, "DO YOU DO COCAINE?"

Now, I probably should have gathered all of this information and come to one conclusion: *Run away, Weezy. Run away right now.*

This should've been sign number one to leave. Instead, I stayed. When it came to coke, I'd dabbled here and there as I was learning the ropes of the elite New York party scene. Cocaine wasn't just a white people's drug like I thought it was. It was the RICH people's drug of choice. I obliged him, and we went into the bathroom together. He poured out lines onto a hand dryer, rolled up a $100 bill, and handed it to me after saying, "Ladies first."

He watched me, laughed at how I started coughing afterward because of how strong it was, and kissed me. I remember feeling so much better after he'd kissed me. He was finally having fun with me! The guy who owned his apartment and traveled to places like Aix-en-Provence or St. Barth for the weekend liked me!

Ol Bae had proven to be too much of a party boy for me, so I kind of left him at the bottom of my texts for a while. But one June night, my breakup with Scissors was haunting me. I hadn't realized how unique and rare my relationship with her was until I dated other people. She was just so fucking special.

Scissors wasn't scared of her feelings, scared to touch me in public, or scared to be clear about how she felt at any given time. Maybe it's because I had been only dating men after her, but even to this day, it is hard for me to have intimacy beyond sex with other women. This is something I really don't care to dig into with my therapist, but it does tend to pop back up in my mind every once in a while.

I texted Ol Bae that I was feeling sad and needed to use him to forget about my sadness. I sat at the bar at Sisters and told him all about my throuple, but especially HER. He suddenly seemed to be more interested in me than he ever was. I could see it all over his face. HMM, a bisexual girl who's sad and already used to having threesomes? GREAT!

Remembering the first time we had sex is a constant ego boost for me because I'd never had a man say what he did that night. We'd started with drinks at Sisters in Brooklyn because it was close to his apartment, and he seemed to discern that tonight would be the night.

When we got back to his place, we had a messy make out, and since it wasn't that great, I decided to go down on him to break up the weird kiss. It had been a while since I'd had a new dick in my mouth. I assume it's as exciting as men say new pussy is to them, but I love giving someone head for the first time.

I know that the biggest difference between myself and many encounters that men say they've had before is that I will suck it like it's my fucking religion. I do it all. I get down on my knees and unzip the pants myself. I smile and do that flirty giggle while I reach my hand to pull his dick through the hole in the boxers. I'm never in a rush. I grab it with one hand while the other is on his thigh. I grip hard but lightly kiss from the shaft all the way to the head, exploring with my mouth. I pay so much attention not just because I listen, but because I'm watching, I'm feeling, and I'm in perfect alignment with his body language.

Turns out I sucked Ol Bae's dick a little TOO good that first time. He was worried about cumming too fast, so he rushed to get a condom from his pants on the floor. Ol' boy was so weak from how good I was sucking him that he pleaded with me to get on top. Usually, before I put a dick inside of me, I do that little swipe of spit on my pussy—mainly because I love having a man watch me lick my fingers and touch myself, but also to make sure I feel hella juicy. I used my right hand to make sure he was going in the right place, got up on my feet, and started to ride him. He was moaning so LOUDLY. It was so loud I almost thought he was faking it.

He stopped me and said, "Listen to me; you are ALWAYS going to fuck me. You hear me? You 'bout to fuck me all the fucking time. This pussy is about to be MY shit. We going to be fucking ALL. THE. TIME."

I'd never had anyone say that. The feeling of being *that* wanted had me looking past a lot of shit. A man in his forties with no real serious relationship history or kids. A man in his forties who's getting high every weekend, known on every party scene, running around with a twenty-seven-year-old ME! HELLO, RED FLAGS.

RED FLAGS I SHOULD HAVE NOTICED

HISTORY OF SHORT-TERM RELATIONSHIPS—A pattern of brief relationships or a reluctance to settle down can be a red flag. If he frequently moves from one relationship to another without forming lasting bonds, it could indicate a fear of commitment.

AVOIDING EMOTIONAL INTIMACY—If he shies away from deeper emotional conversations and keeps things on a superficial level, it can be a sign that he's not ready to form a deeper, committed bond.

PARTYING EXCESSIVELY—If he frequently prioritizes partying and socializing over spending quality time with you, it might indicate a lack of readiness for a committed relationship. Excessive partying can suggest that he values a carefree lifestyle more than building a stable and serious partnership.

I ignored the signs, and over the next few months, we had a crazy-ass love affair. Usually, we'd start with a party and end with sex in his apartment. I would be lying if I said the sex with him alone was amazing, but for sure, it was a fun time. Yet what was more fun were the threesomes with some of the podcast listeners after we walked into Las Lap. Binges and benders with people we met that came back to his place after a night at the elite Soho bar, The Blond. Or just rough sex together after we spent a night at a strip club and were hate-fucking because we didn't take home someone from there.

He never made love to me. He tried, but it wasn't real. I dated him for three years, and I remember feeling like fucking him was always a sport. I knew that many of the threesomes were attributed to him being thirsty for other women, especially considering he treated a night out with me like a night out by himself. Most times, I would find him in the face of another woman by the time I came back from the bathroom. But it's crazy because he always won me over by having a big smile on his face. He knew where my deepest insecurities lay. He never left me feeling left out up until the pandemic. When life slowed down, I felt his energy growing bored with me. After all, we had only connected by doing drugs and partying. What the fuck did we know about being in the house? It's not like our relationship was BAD. It was just *there*.

I had learned his cell phone password after a drunken night the year before when I had to call us an Uber. I'd saved it in my notes: 4147. He said it was the last four digits of his credit card back then. I'd never looked through his phone before, but finding that his energy was off, I decided to snoop in February 2020. I had just gotten back from touring in Detroit when he fell asleep, and finally, I was left alone with his phone. I opened the text threads, and to my surprise, I wasn't one of ten like I thought. I was one of fifty. He had so many women he went back and forth with about sex—some that he had just met, some that he'd only texted his apartment address at 4 a.m.

His best female friend, who he used to house-swap with when he would travel to LA, the girl I thought I was the MOST safe with—he was fuckin' that bitch, too! I was furious. What was even crazier? He sent the days that I was touring as his days of availability to other women. Like clockwork, I'd leave for the airport for a show, and within ten or twenty minutes he was off to the next bitch. The only difference between the bulk of texts I had seen vs. the ones he sent to me was consistency. I was the only woman he consistently chatted with, the only one he initiated a conversation with every day, the only one he expressed love for, and somehow, this pacified me.

I put the phone down, crawled back into bed, and wanted to scream. But I couldn't admit what I had just done. I would look crazy! How would he trust me? Why was I worried about his trust when he had lost mine? Was he using condoms? Was it because we weren't deep enough in love? Maybe he would stop one day. I stayed up another two hours feeling angry and crying at the same time. He slept through it all.

When morning came, he pulled me close to him, kissed me all over, and we had sex. I cried while he fucked me. I didn't cry because I didn't want it; I actually think I came. I cried because I was so disappointed with how I let this man treat me. Since I let that first night go . . . it was hard to bring it up later. One night turned into almost two more years.

I think I also stayed because I had been through far worse when I was younger. When I was just out of high school, I got into a shitty relationship with a man who was ten years my senior and who was abusive as hell. BUT! At least he had money. This was during the time when my dad had lost almost everything due to his business going bust. This man was able to lend some to my family to keep us afloat, buy me expensive things, move me into his home, and hit me whenever he felt like I disobeyed him.

I'd learned to be the illusion of the perfect housewife from my mother. I set the table just so, learned how to cook his favorite meals and have them waiting for him, greeted him at the door, wore his favorite scent, and looked the way he liked me to. The largest difference between this man and the one my mother catered to was that my father was the ultimate MAN. He poured into me about my beauty (inside and out), loved me, and set a high standard for myself with how I was supposed to be treated.

Which was nothing like the little I had decided to accept. There are flashes of terrible memories with my partner. He first showed his signs of rage because I beat him in a Scrabble game. He forced me to continue to play until he won, and when I let him win, he flipped the table and went on a drive. He had to cool down because he wasn't allowed to lose, especially to me. Then there was the time he threw me outside in my underwear. I'd almost made it to a gas station when he drove up in the car behind me to apologize and win me back yet again. And one of my worst memories is the time my mom got on her knees and begged him not to hit me anymore.

I had never flat-out told my mother he was hurting me, but her maternal intuition was strong. She asked me so many times to come back home, but considering my parents' money problems, I didn't want to add more stress to the situation. The fact that he was helping pay their bills, too, made me feel even more inclined to stay.

Not only was he abusive, but he was also a cheater. His final time cheating on me taught me everything I needed to know about how men do or do not pay us respect. He had brainwashed me into believing that my highest goal and only job was to take care of him and the house we lived in. That serving our family should be my main responsibility. After two years of convincing me that work was unnecessary, he fell in love with a beautiful woman who was in school to be a dentist and told me he loved her because of her ambition.

I finally packed up my shit and left him. The lesson that I had learned was that I would never let another man hit me. I didn't think about the parallels with the cheating between my ex and Ol Bae. I didn't know that I deserved more, or that radical happiness could actually exist in any relationship. What I had with Ol Bae was good enough. I mean, he didn't beat me. He was a cheater, but it was just sex. He came back home, so what was I complaining about? I really believed that this bar was high enough.

Then, when COVID swept through New York, I figured . . . he's GOTTA slow down, right?!?

Boy, was I wrong. We had a few good weeks, though. We decided to move to Mexico. I subleased my apartment to a friend, and we headed off to Tulum. We took pictures in the airport in March 2020. It was completely dead, like the zombie apocalypse was upon us. Once we arrived, it was like I finally got the boyfriend I'd always wanted. He was working from home, I was making him three meals a day, and we were running on the beach every morning.

Life and my tan were perfect.

Until the rest of the world found out Tulum was a mask-free haven. He may have been removed from women, but women started to flock to the little town. I forced myself to go out with him even when I was exhausted, in fear he'd fuck someone without me. But then there were nights when I wanted him to leave just so I could catch up on his cheating on his laptop. The second I would hear the door latch, I would run down to check his MacBook, with iMessages popping up in real time. It slowly became my full-on addiction, much like his own sex addiction. He would pretend he was in a workout or running to the store, and I would see his messages with other women.

I spent my days in an endless cycle of anxiety and madness, waiting for him to leave just so I could comb through his latest conquests. I grew so obsessive that when the texts got boring, I moved on to his Google search history.

ESCORTS NEAR ME. ESCORTS NOW.

He would type this shit in while I was fucking sleeping next to him. I was already giving this man sex every day, sometimes twice a day. But it wasn't enough. Ain't no pussy like new pussy.

The most painful moment of all came on the day of our Mexican foursome. The irony of this is that in episode 352 of our podcast, *WHOREible Decisions*, titled "Weezy Had a Foursome," I tell a really funny story about how my current partner and I slept with these lesbians one night in Sayulita and it felt like the thing that drew us together! I never considered that in my last relationship, it was the thing that broke us up.

We had heard there was a new hookah bar in town that played

hip hop, and it would be a bit of a change for us, considering Tulum was pretty much the Ibiza of the Western Hemisphere. As we took our little rental into town, he goes, "Baby, can we get some pussy tonight? Come on, baby! I wanna have some fun with you!"

I was so annoyed with this nigga. Just a few hours before, we'd gotten in a huge fight about a secret call he'd had outside that he swore was his homeboy. I just couldn't stand him. I couldn't even believe the gall that he'd ask me that. I told him to leave me alone and turned up the radio. But was he really all that bad? I would ask myself what he was doing to hurt me besides just being "a guy." Trust me, I know I'm painting this man out to be a piece of shit, but I would always return to the thought that not everything was perfect. I sat in the passenger seat, trying to be grateful for the things about this person that I did love, even if it was as simplistic as the feeling of his hand on my leg as we were heading to explore this beautiful jungle we lived in. That morning, he'd surprised me with a massage because he knew I was working myself out a little too hard. That's the type of man you keep, right? Maybe I was supposed to let the other stuff go? And so, at that moment, I did.

We got into the new spot, and it was kind of popping. We ran into some other Black people we knew from NYC and one of our homeboys out there. He was talking to a group of three girls. They were super cute, from Atlanta, and all of them were nurses. They had such an "I'm on a spring break" vibe about them. Not too young—I would have guessed late twenties. Normally, I can spot a threesome coming, but with this trio, I really didn't see it.

We started sharing shots with them. I was dancing with one cutie in particular, and when the club was starting to close, they asked us where to go next. Before I could tell them everything was shut down, he said, "OUR PLACE!" I remember looking back at him and saying nothing, but it was clear that the look in my eyes said NO. That look a mother gives you when you start touching shit in the grocery store—don't even gotta say shit! He pulled me into the corner and said, "Baby, we're just gonna have fun. We don't even need their names. Let's just have fun, baby."

I don't know why I did it. I think I was so tired of feeling like I had changed in our relationship that it was hard not to go along with the version of me I had created, the woman he fell in love with. Even though love was not actually a part of the equation. Even though I was so mad at him, I still wanted his approval.

We got back to our two-bedroom villa; the girls came in. Our homeboy takes one in the room and the other two come into the master with me. Ol Bae ran to go get condoms, not because anyone discussed what was happening, but mainly because it was 5 a.m.

The girls started to undress and cuddle in the bed, saying how nervous they were. I got naked, and to be quite honest, I felt the same. I didn't know if they were friends or coworkers, but I had a string of thoughts that started to piece together at five in the fucking morning.

I felt one of them push her ass up on me in the bed, and when I didn't give enough of a response, she turned around to me and said, "Are you gay?" I said, "Yeah, I kinda am." She took it upon herself to get on top of me and start kissing me. Her body felt so fucking amazing. I remember how much I enjoyed feeling a woman on me again. I usually don't have a voyeur in the mix, but the other woman watched as we started to make out and lick on each other's nipples.

I turned her over and started eating her pussy from the back. I remember laughing to myself a little bit, thinking about how lucky I was that her pussy tasted so good for being out all night in a sweaty Mexican club. Her friend got tired of watching us and joined in, and we were literally in this sexy-ass pussy-eating triangle. It felt so fucking good, and honestly, I was glad he wasn't there.

I remember making one of them cum from sucking on her clit really, really hard. I'm usually so gentle, but she could handle a lot! She was so fucking sexy, too, the way she kept telling me I wasn't giving it to her hard enough. She was grabbing the back of my head and forcing herself into me so hard I was almost worried I would scratch her with my teeth! We got louder and louder.

When he finally walked in, they were looking forward to it, but my body language changed. He said, "Oh shit, y'all got it popping without me?" He asked me to come outside for a second, and frankly, I didn't even wanna look at him. He told me how he couldn't find condoms, and so he asked me to wake up my best friend Venny, who was visiting from the States and staying in the unit next door.

"Are you fucking kidding me? No," I said. "Just don't have sex, bro. What the fuck are you always so goddamn thirsty for a bitch for? I didn't even wanna do this shit. Now I gotta be on the hunt for your muthafuckin' condoms?!?!?" I started to scream at him in a way that I never had. I remember how he looked at me. He said, "You don't love me anymore, G. Do you?"

I didn't even answer him. He looked like he was about to cry. He asked me what we were supposed to do and how we were supposed to figure this out.

AS IF I CARED.

I walked out, went into Venny's apartment, grabbed condoms, threw them at Ol Bae, and walked back over to spend the night at my friend's place. I silently cried again, just like the night I went through his phone in New York. Silently crying had become my specialty.

It was so clear to me this time. Maybe he was sex-crazed and addicted to pussy before, but this time, he made a definite choice. I left, I walked away, I was in tears, and he chose to turn his back on me and chose his addiction over his girlfriend.

Our relationship took many more months to end. This pain he gave me was easier to deal with when I had him wipe my tears at night than the pain I would've felt without him. A real breakup was worse than just staying with him. I like to think I used him as my stepping stool, a way to feel a little stability while I got my new life together—not stability in the sense of money, but just to not be alone.

During our breakup, I sold my TV show to Fuse, and *WHOREible Decisions* got picked up by the Black Effect Network. Having my own identity helped me not to feel so sad about his addiction to other women. I needed that win on my own to feel like I was better without him. And I was glad he didn't help me to get there. I take so much pride in my success that sometimes it feels like a big FUCK YOU to the men before. I have always felt that there is only one thing a man thinks he can hold over me, and it is and forever will be money.

Our ending was as ridiculous as the way we started. I had always heard the phrase "When shit starts fucked up, it ends fucked up." There was nothing complicated about my decision to leave. However, his reaction was one that I wished I had received that night of the foursome that never was. He was empathetic, remorseful, and even in therapy for his addiction. He finally said all the words I had wanted to hear during the bad times. Below is a line from his last message to me.

He said that he had forsaken me and my love and that he hated himself before finally admitting, "It took me hurting you time and time again to realize how much I'm hurting myself because I have never loved anyone as much as I love you."

By the time the message that I'd been waiting for arrived, it was too late. I had learned not to give up on myself. I knew that I deserved more, and I was giving it to Weezy. I didn't need him or anyone else.

Love, sex, intimacy—it's literally all a drug. The high, the excitement of being in a relationship, even when you *know* it ain't the one for you . . . but you keep going through the motions 'cause, let's be real, it's easier than dealing with a breakup. It's not that bad, right? It's comfortable. Familiar. And breaking up feels like a whole hassle you're just not ready to face.

One of the wildest moments for me while writing about Ol Bae came after a town hall with our podcast listeners. Mandii hit me with a comment that stuck with me for days. She said she was shocked to read all the messed-up things I put up with and how Ol Bae made me feel because I never acted like it was that deep. I always made it seem like it wasn't so bad. And, honestly, hearing that? It hurt. I knew she didn't mean it like that, but it was a reflection of the story I was putting out there. The truth is, I wasn't lying to anyone—I was blinded by love and the comfort of companionship. In real time, I was telling my side, but I was downplaying the pain I was pushing aside, pretending it was just regular relationship struggles.

The thing about relationships that have run their course is that they're the hardest to see for what they really are. It's not always some big "you have to break up" moment. He wasn't mean. He didn't yell. He always paid. He had a good job. He treated me nicely. We had fun. We had a real friendship. So how could I get on my podcast and explain a feeling I couldn't fully comprehend? I kept telling myself, *Aren't all relationships hard? Won't I just have to start over? It's not that bad. It could be worse, right?*

And then it hit me. One day, like any other, I was simply done.

I'm never settling again for being second or third to someone else's addictions. I'm not sticking around for someone who only wants to party through life. I want a partner who can handle the ups and downs with me. And if they can't? I'll navigate this life solo. 'Cause honestly, sometimes the realest, bravest move is choosing to BE SINGLE.

Recognizing that you've stayed in a toxic relationship for too long can be challenging, but there are signs that may indicate it's time to reevaluate the situation.

SIGNS YOU'VE STAYED TOO LONG

LACK OF TRUST—Trust is fundamental in a healthy relationship. If you constantly doubt your partner's intentions or honesty, or if they regularly break your trust, this is a serious red flag.

CONSTANT STRESS AND ANXIETY—If your relationship is a significant source of stress and anxiety rather than a source of support and comfort, it may be toxic.

FEELING DRAINED—A healthy relationship should energize you. If you feel emotionally, mentally, or physically exhausted from the relationship, it's a sign that something is wrong.

FREQUENT CRITICISM—If your partner constantly criticizes, belittles, or undermines you, it can erode your self-esteem and is indicative of a toxic dynamic.

ISOLATION—If your partner tries to isolate you from friends, family, or other support systems, this is a manipulative tactic often used in toxic relationships.

LACK OF RESPECT—Mutual respect is crucial. If your partner consistently disrespects you, your feelings, or your boundaries, it's a major issue.

UNEQUAL EFFORT—Healthy relationships involve both partners putting in effort. If you feel like you are always the one trying to make things work while your partner is indifferent, it can be draining and unfair.

FEAR OF YOUR PARTNER—If you feel afraid of your partner, whether it's fear of physical harm, emotional abuse, or manipulation, it's a clear sign of toxicity.

DISHONESTY AND MANIPULATION—If your partner lies, manipulates, or gaslights you, it can make you doubt your reality and your worth.

INCOMPATIBILITY AND CONSTANT CONFLICT—While all relationships have conflicts, constant fighting or fundamental incompatibilities that lead to regular arguments can be signs that the relationship is unhealthy.

Recognizing these signs is the first step toward taking action to protect your well-being. If you identify with several of these points, it may be beneficial to seek support from friends, family, or a professional.

Patriarchal Bullshit
"When a lady says no, she means maybe,
and if she says yes, she's not a lady."
—Sebastián Piñera (former Chilean president,
close of a summit of heads of state in Mexico in 2011)

Matriarchal Reply
"Men celebrated our sexual liberation—our willingness to
freely give and enjoy blow jobs and group sex, our willingness to experiment with anal penetration—but ultimately
many males revolted when we stated that our bodies were
territories that they could not occupy at will."
—bell hooks (activist and author of
Communion: The Female Search for Love)[1]

WELL, WHAT WERE YOU WEARING?*

« MANDII B »

I JOKINGLY REFER to myself as one of "God's Favorites" because of my three-day period and very light PMS symptoms. I also have a few other superpowers, such as having big-dick radar and the ability to orgasm via penetration. Yup, these things make me one of "God's Favorites," at least in my mind. And above all, I considered myself to be "special" because I had never been sexually violated. I know that sounds wild. I know! But I genuinely felt grateful not to have encountered the traumatic experiences that so many of my peers and loved ones had. According to the CDC, "over half of women and almost one in three men have experienced sexual violence involving physical contact during their lifetimes. One in four women and about one in twenty-six men have experienced completed or attempted rape. More than four out of five female rape survivors reported that they were first raped before age twenty-five and almost half were first raped as a minor."[2] So, because I wasn't part of those horrifying statistics, I felt that I was blessed and highly favored.

It was a breezy November day, and global warming had gotten the best of New York City as it held tight to the grip of the warmer fall weather. I only needed to wear a light jacket to work that morning. At the time, I had a job at Goldman Sachs as I also navigated my final year of college. I was taking seven classes that last semester and was only five months away from graduating with 151 credits, enough to lock in two bachelor's degrees as I prepared for my career in accounting. I didn't have classes on this day, so I worked a quick 11–5 shift, which was normal when we weren't buried in K-1s or dealing with a busy tax season. There was a routine. I worked in Jersey City but lived in the Bronx. From work, I caught the PATH train at Journal Square and took it into Manhattan to the Fulton St./ World Trade Center stop. I would then take the 5 train and transfer at 125th to the 6 express to my neighborhood, Parkchester.

I crammed myself onto the subway with all the other commuters on their way home from a long, tiresome day at work. I had lived in New York for about five years at this point, and this was also pre-COVID, so the idea of personal space as a New Yorker in need of public transportation didn't exist. I boarded the train with the thoughts of plopping down on my couch, having a glass of wine, and catching an episode of *Chopped* to relax. Instead, I'd spend that night fighting with my psyche.

I was among the last people to board, so I stood by the doorway. With my hand above me grasping on to the pole for stability, the doors almost slid closed behind me before one more person shoved their way onto the train. As we rode from the 125th station on the Bronx-bound 6, the last-minute passenger found a way to situate himself closer to me than I deemed necessary. I remember looking back and rolling my eyes as a signal to let him know that he was too close and to BACK THE FUCK OFF. I shoved my laptop bag between us, attempting to use it as a barrier. I knew that this would give any sane person the hint that their proximity felt odd and intentional. At the first stop, the doors opened on the other side of the car, so I remained stuck. I just wanted to get to my place and get away from the sardines-in-a-can feeling that I endured on every commute.

The second stop was even farther away since we skipped so many stations on the express. The ride got extremely bumpy as we rode from 138th to Hunts Point. The train picked up speed, and everyone had to hold on to the poles more tightly as we got jostled about and tried to keep our balance. The man behind me was taking full advantage of the instability in the car and jutting into me from the back even more. I had nowhere to move to and was utterly frustrated with this guy bumping into me over and over again. I assumed he had not been taught the common courtesy of giving another human personal space. Then again, I was on a packed train during rush hour. I told myself I had to work harder to afford a car or a driver, but until then, I'd have to deal.

As we pulled into the Hunts Point stop, I was finally going to be able to get some space and catch my breath because I was by the doors that opened to release passengers. As the doors opened, the man who stood behind me and I both had to step outside onto the platform. I froze as I turned to look at the man who had ignored my hints and attempts at finding personal space. I looked down to see that he had his dick exposed. Our eyes met. I looked down again as he quickly stuffed his half-flaccid penis back into his pants. I was in shock. He broke our stare, turned around, and briskly disappeared into the crowd.

I stood, silent. I stepped back onto the train and began to weep. The train was much less packed now. I was in the exact spot that I'd been standing in with my perpetrator, and I just cried. I'm wiping away tears now as I share this with you. While the tears SHOULD come from the trauma of recounting this violating encounter, they are from the anger that still exists from how I responded at that moment. Or feel like I failed to respond. I cried in front of all these strangers, and I still can't believe how I'd been such a coward.

After hearing so many stories and seeing movies, I had it in my head that I would never find myself in such a compromised position. I had all these ideas about how I would protect myself if I ever needed to. I envisioned fighting back with the same fists I'd used growing up to defend myself. I told myself I'm strong and don't take shit from anyone. I imagined myself making a scene and embarrassing the perpetrator because I was so loud. "YOU PERVERT!" I would scream and alert everyone to the fact that this weirdo had violated me. I even envisioned myself as Leonidas, king of the Greek city of Sparta, from my favorite film, *300*. If I was ever in a scenario where I had to beat off multiple abusers at once, I'd somehow navigate it like a warrior and come out as victor. But I did nothing. I stood there crying instead—a victim.

An older Latina woman in the car looked concerned and asked me if I was okay. Through tears and snot, I remember saying, "That man just rubbed his dick on me this whole ride. I saw it." Other women heard what I said and became concerned. They suggested we take the train back from the next stop and go back to find him. I knew that wasn't an option. He would be long gone by now or riding another train, probably doing to someone else what he had just gotten away with doing to me. The next stop was finally mine. Stop number three, and I exited the train like I did every other day. My mind was moving faster than my thoughts could keep up, and I started to blame myself. Why didn't I switch cars at the first stop?

Why didn't I speak up? Why didn't I punch him? Why was I only able to cry and not scream out?

Then, the strangest thought crossed my mind. One that I still grapple with today. I asked myself, *Why did he have to be Black?* Not that we usually imagine who or what our abuser will look like, but it infuriated me even more that he was a Black man. How could he do this to his sister? A study found that 91 percent of Black women who are assaulted are sexually assaulted by Black men, and 75 percent of those attacks are by men they know.[3] There is already so much trauma associated with our lineage. And even today, we still find our backs against the wall as we fight for equality and against racism and capitalism as a community. Why would this Black man add to my trauma? This is where my mind went. I was battling both rage and pity at the same time while placing a majority of the blame squarely on myself.

I picked up the phone and called a close friend of mine. He was near and dear to me and someone who often made me feel safe. So naturally, he was my first phone call. I shared what had just happened to me. Looking back and conversing with him later, I know he genuinely didn't know how to respond. But in the moment, his awkwardness on the subject led him to blurt out what is said far too often to women. **"Well, what were you wearing?"**

I was stunned. He'd added a sheepish laugh after the question before complimenting me on how big and nice my ass looked. I immediately started to defend myself. I was coming from work. I'd had on a burgundy cardigan over a plain black tank top. My pants were loosely fitted black pants from New York & Company. And my shoes were black flats so hideous that they fit right into my dull work environment. And this was just the first male response I had gotten like this. Similar responses were yet to come.

It turns out that many women find themselves in the same

situation. Most victims do not report sexual violence immediately or at all. The reasons can be complicated, but here are a few:

- The victim **DOESN'T IMMEDIATELY ACKNOWLEDGE OR LABEL THE EVENT AS AN ASSAULT, TRAUMA, OR SEXUAL ABUSE.** They may not even understand that what they went through was rape/sexual assault. Often survivors can't even say the word "rape" out loud for years, especially in reference to their own experience.
- The victim is **AFRAID THEY WON'T BE BELIEVED,** either because the assailant is in a position of power or is well-liked.
- The victim is **WORRIED THEY ARE AT FAULT.** Maybe they had something to drink, initially eagerly engaged in making out, or agreed to go somewhere alone with a person and they think they should have "known better."
- The victim **DOESN'T THINK THEY CAN EMOTIONALLY HANDLE IT** if their attacker is found "not guilty" or "not responsible." This is a tough one, because it's a realistic fear.
- The victim feels that reporting won't make a difference because it **CAN'T ERASE THE TRAUMA.**

I also figured that there was nothing I could do. The event happened. I wouldn't seek justice, and I had to move on! I dealt with this in silence. While I brought up what had happened to my mom and my friends, I was met with condolences and "I'm sorrys," but nobody had died, and what the fuck were they even apologizing for? I didn't feel like anything or anyone could help me, so in typical

Mandii fashion, I decided to bury it. I figured I'd come back and deal with it later, as I do with too many things that leave me feeling uncomfortable.

A few weeks later, I found myself as a guest on a podcast with Liris Crosse, a plus-sized model I had the joy of learning about during her time on *Project Runway*. We had both agreed to be guests to discuss fat-shaming, dating as a plus-sized girl, and the objectification of women's bodies. The podcast host was a straight cis male who cosplayed as an ally to women's plights. At the time, I viewed this man as a friend. We were both navigating the new podcasting landscape; he had just lost his co-host. I agreed to assist him with this new creative pivot and looked forward to participating in this conversation.

I sat in my black Duke hoodie across from the stunning Liris Crosse, who sported a "Curvy By Nature" T-shirt. There was one camera to capture the video and three mics for each of our stories. I'm not sure which topic led me to open up about my recent sexual assault, but I bared my soul and illustrated the horror of my train ride from work. I cried and shared about my assault. It didn't bother me that a stranger was in the room because she was a woman. She shared so many of the same experiences as me, navigating trying to find clothes that fit, battling the scale and self-worth, and taking on society's views on women who aren't a size six.

I thought this would be a safe space with a man I believed to be a friend. His first question as I dried my tears after spilling my heart out was "Well, shouldn't you expect to be sexually assaulted?" At the moment, I felt like this was just another man not knowing how to handle a woman opening up about an assault who spoke without thinking. I was confused. "Excuse me? WHAT?" I wanted to be sure he wasn't asking for shock value and truly wanted me to answer the question.

He meant what he'd said. He explained how I have a podcast about sex and that as part of my journey and being sexually liberated, I should EXPECT sexual assault. How could I have had a podcast called *WHOREible Decisions*, embracing whoredom, while not expecting men to believe that they had the right to take advantage of me? Here I was, thinking I was being brave and vulnerable and leading the charge in getting more women to feel free to demand what they want from men and their sexual experiences. In my mind, I was positively impacting lives through my own tales of womanhood and sharing how I was navigating life. Instead, according to this man and probably many others, I was wearing a sign inviting men to sexually assault me and violate my boundaries.

What had I done to deserve losing my place as one of "God's Favorites"? Why would God bring this into my life after twenty-seven years and leave me with this trauma? Was my modern approach to sexual freedom opening up the possibility of this happening to me again? Would I be able to fight back next time? Must there be a next time?

I thought that maybe if this had happened to me when I was younger, I would have known how to respond as an adult. Well, that turned out to be a foolish thought. If we can't physically protect ourselves from our abusers, somehow, our brain goes into overdrive to shelve the things that could harm us. With many traumatic experiences, a common defense mechanism includes completely forgetting the memories.

It was the summer of 2022, and we were returning to normalcy from the pandemic. Earlier that year, my mom had gotten COVID, and she was so sick that it was a battle we were afraid she'd lose. Fortunately, my mom beat the virus that had taken so many lives in such a short time. I'd never considered losing a parent up until I almost did. This brought about a new fear for me. I understand that everyone will die at some point, but it wasn't until that incident that I imagined a life without my mom. This had to be the same for my sister because now, if one of us calls my mom and she doesn't pick up her phone, we call each other to ask the last time we spoke to her.

As I sat on the train heading to my studio, I looked down at a phone call from the Orange County Sheriff's Department. I was underground and couldn't answer. I immediately got a voicemail notification. Although I didn't have the service to take a phone call, I could play the message. A stern-sounding white man with little emotion introduced himself as a detective in Orange County looking to speak to Amanda Rogers. My heart sank. I texted my mom immediately, asking where she was. It was a Saturday, so she would usually be at work. She had just gotten out of an abusive relationship with a narcissist from hell, and my mind went to flashes of every Lifetime movie I'd ever watched where the man turns into a psycho killer. With no response, I reached out to my sister. "Alex, when was the last time you heard from Mommy? Can you call her?" I continued frantically texting the two of them. I needed to know they were okay. I still had two more stops before I would have service. My sister was responding, but I had not yet heard from my mom. My heart beat out of my chest as I prepared to hear the worst.

I ran to the top of the stairs and tried to catch my breath. I pulled my phone out and called the number left by the detective. He answered. He asked again if I was Amanda Rogers, to which I responded, "Yes." I asked him if everything was okay, and he said he was working on a case and had come across my name in an old file. He said I had been listed as a witness of a sexual crime in 1997 involving an individual who was facing a lot of time for doing something horrible. The details were scant, but my heart rate lowered and I could breathe again. I told him he must have me confused with someone else. I had never been to court and was not a witness to any crimes. I even laughed and said, "Sir, in 1997, I would have been six or seven years old." He then asked about an address I had previously lived at and even knew my mom's and sister's full names. Although he had all this information, I was still convinced this was a mistake.

I asked him to explain the police report he'd referenced with all my information. After confirming more of my details, he began reading the report. He brought me back to my childhood in the most surreal way. As he recounted the words from the report, I was transported to my six-year-old self. My sister and I were playing in the kid's room at my babysitter's house. Dee was her name, and she was a close friend of my mom until she went behind her back and fucked my daddy. When my mom would work, we would stay with Dee. The room was painted an eggshell white that eventually was stained yellow due to all the cigarettes Miss Dee smoked. My sister and I were playing with toys when we heard someone at the window. We were both startled to see a man who had been standing outside of the window watching us play. He smiled and waved for us to come over to the window. Out of innocence, we complied. As we neared the window, he backed up, sat on some concrete cinder blocks that divided her home from the street, and began pleasuring himself. With his pants down to his knees and his bare ass on the bricks, he stroked his dick in front of us.

I didn't know what was happening, but it didn't seem right. I quickly hopped down from the window and went to tell Miss Dee that a man was at our window and his pants were down. She called 911 and quicker than I can even remember, the cops arrived. I had seen cops and the flashing lights before. My sister and I never spoke to cops, but they had come to get Daddy more than once before when he had been mean to Mommy. I snapped out of it as the detective continued to read the words from my six-year-old lips. Here was this stranger, reminding me that I had been sexually violated as a child. A memory pushed so far back into my mind that I forgot it had even happened. I had called myself "God's Favorite" for having not experienced the exact thing that I had removed from the mental archive of my life.

I got ahold of my mom shortly after I hung up with the detective, and she had the same reaction I did. She immediately remembered the day and what had happened, but we both realized it was something that was never brought up or discussed. I recall being told he was a sick, evil man and he wouldn't be at that window anymore. I remember getting the "don't talk to strangers" speech and having to let an adult know if an adult man made me feel uncomfortable. But that was the end of that. I'd sincerely thought I'd gone twenty-seven years unscathed by sexual assault until that moment on the train. Then, at thirty-one, I was reminded of an event when I was only six. The American Psychological Association says, "Women are typically exposed to more interpersonal trauma than men, and often at a younger age. Twenty-five percent of girls experience this form of abuse during childhood."[1] I am a part of that statistic.

Through conversations on the podcast and gaining knowledge around language, I was made aware that I had experienced yet another type of sexual assault by two different men. One was a young NBA player in his second year in the league, and the other was a well-known bad boy in the NFL in his prime. I learned about stealthing on the show and realized it had happened to me in instances with both men. Stealthing is the act of removing a condom during sex without the other person's consent or lying about having put one on. It's a form of rape and reproductive coercion, which is defined as a threat or act of violence against a partner's reproductive health or reproductive decision-making. Twelve percent of women have experienced stealthing, and ten percent of men have admitted to non-consensual removal of a condom, according to a study published by the Jacobs Institute of Women's Health.[5] Though we had agreed to have consensual sex, both men chose to remove their condoms without my knowledge. They both tried to use the excuse of how good my pussy felt and how they wanted to feel all of it.

The NFL player had convinced me to be blindfolded. I hadn't done that before that point, but there was a first time for everything. He took his time eating my pussy. He went from my pussy, up to my breasts, before kissing me and going back down. He kept reiterating to me that I couldn't look. After a while, it was my time to please him. I removed the blindfold and felt him grow inside of my mouth. He was bigger than I thought he'd be, and as he pushed his dick deeper into the back of my throat, I choked. He liked that. I was ready. It was time for him to get inside of me, and I begged him to fill me up with his girthy dick. He ripped open a gold-wrapped condom, and I watched in amazement as he stretched it enough to fit the eight inches he was packing. He got on top and began sensually fucking me. We kissed and he fucked me with a passion that was weird because this was our first time having sex. We changed into a few positions before he asked me to put the blindfold back on. I obliged.

The sex, from what I remember, was great. It felt good. However, the thing I remember most about it was the end. I felt him pulse and moan in ecstasy as he came. He quickly placed his hands over my mask. I giggled and told him "that was fun" as I went to move his hands so that I could remove the blindfold. He stopped me and said, "You're gonna be mad at me."

He had just made me cum, and our first time was exhilarating. I couldn't understand why or how I would be mad at him now. I removed my blindfold and looked at him, sitting on his knees between my legs. His dick was bare. He looked at me and said how it just felt so good and was so wet that he needed to feel all of it and let me know that he had removed the condom. Even worse, there was no visible cum. He hadn't pulled out. Without any family planning conversations and only knowing my full name and birth date because he had purchased my flight just the day before, this man had chosen to bust all up in me. I couldn't believe it.

We spent the next day on Ocean Drive and ran into the Walgreens on South Beach to get the Plan B I requested. I was leaving the next day and would no longer wait to take it. I made him pay for the pill, and when I went to leave the following day, I was surprised to see he had left me a check for $1,000 in his foyer. I felt like this was his way of apologizing, knowing he had fucked up and hoped it would be enough for me not to make a fuss. It was. I remember immediately going to put the check into my account, and once it cleared, I told him thank you. (I *thanked* him.)

Outside of being angry, I never brought this back up to him, despite running into him on numerous occasions in the New York club scene. I didn't bring it up to the other guy, either. I didn't know until years later that what they had both done to me was considered sexual assault. As of 2018 stealthing is punishable as a form of sexual violence in some countries, such as Germany[6] and the United Kingdom.[7] In the U.S., California became the first state to make it illegal to remove a condom without explicit consent in 2021.[8] Stealthing is classified as a civil offense in California rather than a crime, and victims can sue perpetrators directly in civil court.

I'd flitted around, believing I was blessed, lucky, and one of the scarce number of women who would never have to experience or deal with the trauma of sexual assault in their lifetimes. I honestly had not felt the trauma of being violated until that day on the train, not realizing this wasn't the first time. The previous times I had been violated, I was protected by my youth and ignorance. As a six-year-old, I didn't know a man jacking off in front of my playroom window was an assault. At eighteen and twenty-four, I'd chosen to have protected, consensual sex with these millionaire athletes and had no clue that the removal of a condom would later be cited as a sex crime.

Perhaps this is why I am so adamant now about consent and having multiple conversations with someone before engaging in anything sexual. I find it challenging to be blindfolded in any setting. I wait for the next train if one seems too packed.

At thirty-three, I am still trying to work through my sexual assault experiences. I am trying to make sense of it all while making sure that my past doesn't bleed into and ruin my current relationships with men. I only want to be and have only ever been with Black men. So, despite having these negative experiences with Black men, I still truly believe I can and will have a healthy relationship in and out of the bedroom with a Black man. I want a healthy sex life, and more than ever, I try to be as vocal about the things that I do and do not wish in the bedroom. I firmly believe that God doesn't give us anything he doesn't feel we can handle. I've survived and will only continue to thrive because nothing I have had to overcome will break me, and none of these men can take that power given to me. I've had to reconcile and change my definition of what "God's Favorite" means, but I still know that I am.

RAINN

If you or someone you know has been sexually assaulted, help is available at Rainn.org/resources.

RAINN (Rape, Abuse & Incest National Network) is the nation's largest anti–sexual violence organization. RAINN created and operates the National Sexual Assault Hotline in partnership with more than one thousand local sexual assault service providers across the country.

They have a telephone hotline as well as online chat resources in English and Spanish.

Patriarchal Bullshit

"I'm automatically attracted to beautiful women—
I just start kissing them. It's like a magnet. Just kiss.
I don't even wait. When you're a star, they let you do it.
You can do anything. Grab 'em by the pussy.
You can do anything."
—Donald Trump (45th and 47th president)[1]

Matriarchal Reply

"Men are afraid that women will laugh at them.
Women are afraid that men will kill them."
—Margaret Atwood (novelist, poet, and literary critic)[2]

DO YOU REALIZE YOU RAPED ME?*

« WEEZYWTF »

WHEN I FIRST started working on this, I thought, *Weezy is gonna be Weezy. I'm going to find a way to make this rape story funny.* Obviously, now I know this was a defense mechanism kicking in. That should've been all the warning I needed, wanting to sugarcoat something that is *not* fucking funny. When I got into it, instead of it being funny, I became paralyzed. I couldn't write. Thirteen years after the fact, I couldn't type. The joke was still on me.

I genuinely want to share this story because, although Google states that one in four women have been assaulted,[3] the number sure seems higher within my circle of friends, colleagues, and even my mother. But what makes this story awkward for me to share is that one of my biggest fantasies is rape.

I have heard people call it "consensual nonconsensual sex," but that's just because the R-word is very triggering. In reality, it is what it is. I want my partner to come through my door forcefully, rip my clothes off, pin me to the bed, and enter me while I'm screaming. It literally makes me wet just thinking about it. There's even a part of me that wants to be slapped, gagged, bound by the wrists, just to feel fucking used. My porn history has always been demented. Even at sixteen, I was watching punishment and humiliation videos. No, I didn't have some childhood trauma that made me this way; I'm just a nasty woman! As an adult, I realized that all my recent searches fit under the umbrella of my love of being a submissive:

Bukkake
Black girl punished spanking
Extreme gagging
Public humiliation walked on leash
Human furniture

I feel ashamed that my kink for being dominated goes to the lengths of rape, but I also can't shame myself for it. I can want a fantasy to take place with a safe and trusted person! There is NOTH-ING wrong with reclaiming my sexuality, no matter how someone has taken advantage of me. To be honest, more than therapy has helped . . . The way that I think about myself and talk to myself changed. I have always been a sexual person, and I wasn't gonna let some fucking asshole strip me of my own pleasures.

However, after years of healing, I thought I'd talked this through. I have an understanding that niggas are just sometimes . . . DUMB. People make mistakes. I've forgiven him. Yet, just because we are healed doesn't mean we forget. There's never going to be an easy way to tell a story so beyond hurtful and disgusting about the most violating thing that's ever happened to me. So I'm just going to try.

In 2011, I wasn't even twenty-one yet, but I was running the streets. I always had a craving for the party. That was where I could dance and connect with people in a way that was beyond conversation. Dancing is one of my favorite things to do.

As I've said, my mother was the ultimate Studio 54 girl; she's lived the life we've seen in documentaries for decades. They say the party gene can be hereditary, but, in our case, it's hoe-reditary. It's essential to know my lil' socialite lineage because I find that it's often the rebuttal used when people are empathizing with a rapist.

"Well, you went out that night . . ."

"You shouldn't have been drinking."

"Well, what were you wearing?" (Shout-out to Mandii's chapter.)

How does my going out and living my life the way that I want to become an excuse for someone to rape me? Partying too much can definitely increase the chances of a few things: dry skin, faster aging, or a higher body count. But rape?! This should be the one thing that we all unequivocally understand is wrong; our bodies are our own. If we can't agree on this . . .

I met *The Asshole* a year before. I paid an entry fee to see him and his bandmates at a club called Vain in Orlando. I'm not saying I had groupie energy; I had no idea my night would turn into hanging with them. We all had a good time. My roommate got one of the other guys' numbers, and I got his. We did a little MDMA and danced before we headed out for the night. I wasn't fully prepared to sleep with him. One-night stands were not really my thing. I figured keeping the pussy to myself would guarantee a second meetup, right?

A few weeks later, I was on a Southwest flight to Atlanta. I'm unsure if this was my first time getting flown out, but I remember feeling important. I was only going to be there for twenty-four hours, so clearly, it was just sex.

He picked me up, we shared a kiss, and we headed straight to the studio. Now, young and dumb twenty-year-old me thought it was special when, in reality, this dude just went about his regular day while I was there in the background. I got really high off some tree and mingled with the other people in the spot until he was wrapped.

We headed to dinner, where I thought we'd have this fantastic first date together, but nothing went beyond the surface. I was a little bit disappointed, but I knew how to turn around almost any situation. That's the magic of my lineage. So, what happens next? Ecstasy, of course. We spent the next hour laughing hysterically, feeling on each other. I saw my first cross-dresser ever that night at a sex club we went to. I was in my element.

We ended the night with some sweet and sensual sex at his loft, and by morning, I was back in Orlando. That part is shocking, right? You were waiting for me to get into how he raped me. No. That is not how this particular story goes. And that is why I was even more thrown off when the assault happened.

Communication dwindled, as is expected when you are just living your life. His band was doing well, and they were at the point where it seemed like they might blow up. They had a hit song being played on the radio.

We hadn't talked for months when my roommate saw that he had a club appearance coming up in Tampa. I was working at the White House Black Market in the mall then, so I rushed to close up my store that night. We grabbed a bunch of pizza from Sbarro and hopped our silly asses in the car. I was looking forward to seeing him again.

We arrived late, so he and I did not have much interaction—just a few drinks and a little twerk. I don't recall anything notable happening; it just felt like another night in a club. They performed, and of course, a lot of girls were flirting with all the guys in the group.

As the night was ending, *The Asshole* asked me to go back to his room with him. I obliged happily. I was there because I wanted to be around him. And having seen other ladies vying for his attention and knowing he picked me, I can't lie—I felt like I'd won a prize.

We drove behind their tour van and arrived at what was probably an Embassy Suites or something. I do remember telling him that I was very drunk and that I was starting to not feel well. He put his arm around me and said "Chill, shawty," so I did, and we went up to his room.

He started rolling up, and after a few minutes, I realized that I was actually super nauseous. I felt fucking terrible. Now, here's the part where shit gets weird. And by weird, I mean disgusting and incomprehensible.

He told me to jump into the shower so that I would feel better and then to come to bed. Once I got into the bathroom and turned on the shower, I tried to use it as a decoy to cover up the sound of my vomiting. I was on my knees, huddled over the toilet, holding my hair back with one hand and bracing against the bowl with the other.

THIS was when he ENTERED ME for the first time.

I thought he'd come into the bathroom to make sure I was good. I tried to laugh it off because, of course, I was embarrassed. No one wants to be sick in front of a guy they are getting to know and kind of like. He came up behind me to do what I thought was the courtesy check-in. But instead, he forced himself inside of me. I was kneeling down over a toilet full of vomit, and he stuck his dick inside of me.

His HARD dick.

In a room filled with the odor of puke. Let's remember, I'd had pizza on the way to the show. It looked like chunks of blood and smelled like vodka. It was revolting.

I asked him, "What are you doing?" He wouldn't speak to me.

He just kept pushing himself into me. What makes this whole moment weirder for me is that I vividly remember thinking, *This is how I thought the night would end, right? Not the sickness—the sex. If I was going to end up fucking him anyway, am I being dramatic for saying no?*

I held on to each side of the bowl, almost trying NOT to keep throwing up so that I didn't turn HIM off. Imagine that? Being fucked over toilet water and confused about whether or not you were wasting a man's time just by being there. There were no talks about consent during this time. My mom had always taught me what to do if a stranger came on to me, and my father had taught me how to punch, but what prep did anyone give me if I found myself hovering over my last meal? Did I technically consent since I was in his room already? What about this circumstance? Was it my own fault?

The particular details of how I was finally able to break away from him, stand up, get out of the bathroom, and go to the other side of his hotel room are fuzzy. I know I ran across to the window. It was already lifted up because he'd been smoking, and I ran there so that I could continue to throw up.

The Asshole jumped over the bed. I remember this because of the thud on the floor when he landed. I imagined that I knew what a trapped animal must feel like because I couldn't get away; I was puking my guts out, and he continued to violate me. I was now throwing up, ten or so floors up from a parking lot, with this dude fucking me from behind.

I have these two very specific odd memories from that part of the night:

1. BET was blaring on the TV, and "I'm Real" by J.Lo with Ja Rule was playing the remix, and all I could think was *This bitch cannot sing.*

2. There were hundreds of girls in the club begging to go home with him, and he really chose to fuck someone who was throwing up over a windowsill. What a fucking weirdo!

I was floating. I came in and out of my own body multiple times, and finally, after saying NO for what felt like a lifetime, I pleaded and said, "Okay, okay, let me just go to the bathroom one more time, and I'll be back."

He let me go, and I ran to the bathroom. I looked in the mirror to figure out how to get out of this. I knew that I was close to the room door. There was a tall T-shirt on the bathroom floor. I grabbed it, threw it on, and fucking darted for the door and toward the elevator. I ran so fucking fast that I spit up a little bit on the way. I pressed the down button a hundred times. I wasn't sure where I thought I was going, but I knew that anywhere was better than where I'd just been.

The glass doors slid shut right as he ran up behind me. I'd made it in safely, but I could still see him. It felt like I was living in a fucking horror movie. It was terrifying. Right as I was about to turn my body away, I saw him slip on something: it was literally my throw-up.

The elevator descended, and I made it into the lobby. A woman was working behind the counter. I can't imagine my state because she looked at me as if I were the monster in this story. I stood there barefoot in just a T-shirt, and I begged her for help. I told her that he was hurting me. I can't remember if I full-on used the word "RAPE" or not, but I 100 percent remember saying "PLEASE HELP ME." It was like she couldn't hear me. Like I was still behind the glass of the elevator. I was crying and hysterical, and then suddenly, *The Asshole* was next to me again. I froze, but the tears kept flowing.

He explained to her that I was just drunk. I don't know why, but she let him take me back up the elevator and into his room. Maybe she didn't want any trouble. Maybe her shift was almost over. Maybe she thought this young drunk slut deserved what she got. I will never know the answer.

This part of the story almost bothers me the most. If I saw a young woman who needed my help, I would not hesitate to try to help them. There have been times I've stopped to check on random women on the street who are crying next to some hulking dude. I would never have allowed *The Asshole* to take me away. But she did.

On the way up the elevator, he said the same thing, "CHILL, SHAWTY. YOU TRIPPIN'. YOU JUST TRIPPIN'." Back in the room, he was so fucking livid that he told me to lie down and sleep it off. There was no escape at this point, and I was so frightened that I did what he told me. I just prayed that he would leave me alone. I lay as still as possible for the next six or so hours while he slept. This was before Uber and other apps that would've allowed me to get the fuck out quietly without calling a taxi and waking my perpetrator.

The next morning, he was angry when he left. I thanked fucking God that he did so without trying anything else. After the door slammed, I dressed as fast as possible, gathered my stuff, and headed home. Doing a walk of shame that should've never been mine.

I was in complete fucking shock. I couldn't believe this had happened with someone I'd previously had consensual sex with. The bitch behind the counter had treated me like a lamb for the slaughter. I could not comprehend any of it.

Every sixty-eight seconds, an American is sexually assaulted.[4] Every sixty-eight seconds. Start counting to sixty-eight right now and think about the fact that this is an actual statistic from RAINN, the nation's largest anti–sexual violence organization.

I was surprised when I heard that sexual violence is most often perpetrated by someone a survivor knows.[5] In my case, I'd slept with *The Asshole* before, and it was fine and I thought that was how it would continue to be. But I learned that there is no way of knowing.

Sexual violence could occur with your long-term partner. With your husband or wife. No matter what term is used or how the relationship is defined, it is never okay to engage in sexual activity without someone's consent. That's what it comes down to, RIGHT?

IT IS **NEVER** OKAY TO ENGAGE IN SEXUAL ACTIVITY WITHOUT SOMEONE'S CONSENT.

I didn't run to report the assault, either. I wanted to forget. After trying to write this, I am pretty sure that I have PTSD about the situation. Even today, only 25 out of every 1,000 rapists will end up in prison. Only 2.5 percent of people will pay for what they did.[6] And for every Black woman who reports a rape, at least fifteen Black women don't.[7] Maybe my not reporting it makes me part of the problem, but I didn't think anyone would believe me at the time.

Guess what? I ran into *The Asshole* one more time, and he didn't understand that I was mad at him. So I told him what had happened, and he stated I was crazy. He said, "You're trippin'." Like I made it up in my head.

I confronted the other bandmates and told them what happened. They acted like they were in shock, and I remember their faces. One went into another room and spoke to someone else on the phone. Another one of them alluded to it not being the first time they'd heard something like this about him, and that made me feel even more disgusted but slightly better. Like, okay, maybe this was HIS sickness? It made it easier to believe me now, right? Or did everyone think you were a fucking liar because he was a famous person?

The older I've gotten, the more I remember not knowing what to say about my rape. I pushed it to the back of my mind and am only digging it out for you now, and I still don't know what to say about it.

Going back to the top of this chapter: I thought I'd forgiven him.

I owe this man nothing, and I do not have to forgive him.

The fact that I forgive myself . . . This would be the only thing that would matter. But why in the fuck am I forgiving MYSELF for my own RAPE?

How about this instead?

I'm going to forgive SOCIETY for blaming me for my rape. Fuck that, I'm not gonna forgive that. I'm going to ASK society to DO BETTER. I'm going to ask you to listen to a victim quietly without asking them what part they may have played in their own assault.

There would be no point in my suffering through recounting this unless I gave you some practical advice I didn't receive. That's one thing I've learned from doing *Decisions, Decisions*: we talk about topics so that we can bring you possible solutions. Because, yeah, when I'm talkin' on the mic, it's EASY for me to help someone. (Not like the bitch who watched me at the front desk in the tee with no shoes, but ACTUALLY help.)

I could spend hours telling you and everyone I know about prevention steps, how to make a report, and how to ask for help, but I absolutely couldn't advocate for MYSELF. And that's the real tea, ain't it? We are born to care for everyone but our own goddamn selves. Just thinking about it makes me so angry—how much I can do for others but not ME. How many times have I given advice that I know is true, but I can't take for myself?

"BLOCK HIM, GIRL."

"JUST IGNORE HIS CALLS."

"GET A NEW MAN."

Yet I have drowned in my own poor choices. The one poor choice I chose NOT to make was skipping this chapter.

I even called Charlamagne about my reservations, since this book is on his imprint. He answered the phone per usual: "PEACE, MY NIECE!" A very heartwarming thing to hear, considering I actually have no living uncles.

I told him about everything you just read, except I let him know exactly who it was. He was empathetic, of course, and apologized for what happened to me. Finally, I said, "But someone's gonna think I'm telling this story for clout, right?"

And the question that came out of his mouth dictated this chapter.

"WHY ARE YOU WORRIED ABOUT HIM?"

And that is what I want to leave any victim of abuse with. WHY THE HELL ARE WE WORRIED ABOUT THE PEOPLE WHO HURT US?

I know that at the beginning of this, I intended to make this funny, but I failed. However, I would like to get out the funniest part of this scenario—for me, at least.

I googled his net worth . . . and THAT was laughable.

PROGRESSION

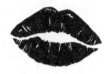

You can only progress with the knowledge learned
from experiencing both pleasure and pain.

Progression is the ultimate goal. Growth requires patience, self-reflection, and perseverance, whether personal, professional, or emotional. We unlock our potential and develop new skills when we lean into discomfort and push beyond our current limits. Embracing the growth process rather than focusing on outcomes allows us to evolve and progress. Through this journey, we open ourselves to new opportunities, gaining deeper insights and reaching new heights, both in our lives and in how we can impact the world around us.

Progression is hard as fuck, but progression is the key to evolution.

Patriarchal Bullshit
"The words and works of God are quite clear, that women
were made to either be wives or prostitutes."
—Martin Luther (NOT KING)
(German priest and theologian)[1]

Matriarchal Reply
"Housework is not work. Sex work is not work.
Emotional work is not work. Why? Because they don't
take effort? No, because women are supposed to provide
them uncompensated, out of the goodness of our hearts."
—Jess Zimmerman (writer and editor)[2]

WHAT'S YOUR PRICE?

« MANDII B »

WHAT WOULD BE the price tag on your pussy? No, seriously. Think about it. The conversations around transactional sex and relationships have become all too much the norm with the red pill topics and ideology across podcasts and social media. We say we want to dismantle the patriarchy, yet have found ways to lean into and uphold it for our own selfish reasons. Turning to "the oldest profession" is commonplace when seeking love, partnerships, and romance. Rudyard Kipling, the originator of the phrase, began his 1889 story about a prostitute with the line, "Lalun is a member of the most ancient profession in the world."[3] Progressives in the early 1900s debated how to address prostitution in the United States, and medical professionals began to cite and also misquote Kipling, giving the phrase a life of its own.

Humans have bartered their bodies for money and goods for thousands of years. If you look back in history, as a society develops material wealth, very shortly after, they create some form of prostitution. While there is constant debate around how much a man should spend on a first date or what gifts a man purchases for a woman they are pursuing, more and more women are blurring the lines between prostitution and romance.

I had very little knowledge about sex work. Growing up in Orlando, I saw streetwalkers prancing up and down Orange Blossom Trail with their miniskirts and platform heels, waiting for anyone to stop and show interest. I was privy to the girls who posed nude in magazines like *Penthouse* and *Playboy*. While in high school, one of my friends worked as a stripper at Magic City. But I had zero intel on the going rates, why these women chose this lifestyle, and how they were introduced to such a life. Of all the careers, why this one? How much money did they make? Where did they find the guys willing to spend the money? It was all a mystery to me.

Well, remember when I said that your environment has a significant impact on your sexual journey and the things you may experience along the way? This is where my early visions of relationship dynamics and finances strongly impacted my views as an adult. My mom left home at fifteen due to the abusive nature of her stepdad. Years later, she saw the relationship between her mother and stepfather fall apart, leaving her mom with absolutely nothing and having to start from scratch.

This pushed my mom to be independent and in control of her financial freedom while being overly protective of the men she allowed to be around us growing up. Unfortunately, her independence and deep-rooted traumas made her the perfect target for men who could take advantage of her. My mom didn't like asking men for anything, nor did she expect them to do much. I assume it's because she had never received these acts of love from men. I saw my mom become the caregiver and provider to grown-ass men who helped very little around the household. These men, over time, would show their true colors. They were cheaters, manipulators, and emotional and financial abusers.

Seeing the behavior of taking care of a grown man as a shortcoming growing up, I vowed never to care for a man financially. We've all heard the saying now: "Why cry in a Honda when you can cry in a Rolls-Royce?" Once again, my father devalued his role in our lives to that of just a human ATM. He would constantly remind us that he paid my mother child support, and so he was doing his part. I can't recall an entire conversation with my dad that involved him having any advice or answers for what I struggled with. I grew up around a man with very limited emotional intelligence. His ability to make money and provide was all he needed to feel like a man, which is also what I believed mattered.

I moved away from home just two days after graduating high school. As I already told you, I packed up my 2002 Hyundai Sonata and drove north for six hours to reunite with Atlanta. Having zero concept of real money and thinking I was ready for adulting, my account was stacked with a whopping $1,800. I'd saved up from my retail jobs at Rue21 and Coach and had gotten my first decent tax return that year. But the alternator blew in my car on my drive to freedom and adulthood. About two hours away from Orlando, I had to sink or swim. I found an AutoZone in the middle of Gainesville and begged a mechanic to take the job immediately. This ended up running me $400, so by the time I reached my final destination, I had less than $1,400 to my name.

I stayed with a friend of mine and his parents when I arrived, but I was adamant this would be temporary. Within a month, I had two jobs—a stock manager position at Diesel and a representative at a call center—and moved into an income-stabilized apartment. I found myself working forty-plus hours and still barely making enough to purchase a bed and settle into my new place. I'd spend most of my hours at work and the leftover hours with friends, new and old. Between the fast life of Atlanta and the circle I found myself a part of, my friends became a blend of celebrities' children, video vixens, porn stars, and girls like me, just trying to figure out how to survive.

In my late teens and early twenties, I didn't fit society's image of a woman who would be pampered by celebrities or attend the hottest parties in the city. I stood at 5'1" and my weight would fluctuate between 180 and 200 pounds, but I had reached 230 pounds at my biggest size. I wasn't laced with the finest designer threads and barely knew how to apply drugstore strip lashes. I was curvy, opinionated, and outspoken, but far from the women you'd see in the magazines and music videos. I was not always the prettiest in my friend groups or the baddest at the table in the club. However, I had confidence and was a hell of a good time. I found myself bagging men I hadn't thought would look past certain women to see me. From athletes to diplomats to rappers, there isn't a one-size-fits-all mold for what people like. One of the men who put me on payroll during college met me when I stood behind a bar in Applebee's sporting all-black pants and nonslip Skechers while serving up Bahama Mamas and sangrias. I remember being shocked to gain the attention of one of the most famous and beautifully chiseled rappers from the early 2000s one weekend in Miami. Confidence is often sexier and more desirable than a woman who is insecure and shy. Men genuinely love an outgoing attitude, even if they don't know it isn't real.

An article from *The Atlantic* describes survival sex as a form of prostitution engaged in by people because of their extreme need.[*] This can include trading sex for food, a place to sleep, or other basic necessities. And according to a write-up in *Teen Vogue* published in

2016, researchers have estimated that one in three homeless youth in North America have engaged in survival sex.[5] And with soaring rents that exceed the average yearly income, more people are finding themselves having to use sex as a means to afford a roof over their heads. Because of the negative connotations around the word "prostitute," many people engaging in these relationships may not even consider themselves as participants in sex work.

I vividly remember my first go at what I would consider sex work. My friend, who was a porn star, hit my line and invited me on a trip. She had explained how it would be with an NBA player from the Cleveland Cavaliers, but we would be going to Phoenix, Arizona, for a weekend turn-up. She let me know that they were looking for a group of "fun" girls and that we would each get paid $1,000 for our attendance. Flights and rooms would be covered, and we just had to "have a good time." I knew there was a possibility of sex, but that didn't faze me. After all, I'd had sex with men for much less. I was sleeping on an air mattress and saw this as my way to get ahead.

The first night was awkward. There were five of us; for whatever reason, one girl was completely blindsided by what sort of trip she had been invited on. She was in tears before the men even joined us for the evening. I tried to tell her how it wouldn't be so bad, even though I'd never done anything like this. She was put on the very next flight back home. I don't remember much from that first night besides getting really drunk and lying on the bed as my friend got fucked at the end of it. I watched her as I zoned in and out. I woke up the next morning, having been unfucked, and thought, *Well, that was easy.*

The next day, we went to Buffalo Wild Wings for lunch, where I agreed to eat ten of the hottest wings on the menu for a pot in the middle of the table that had accumulated $600. Little did they know that the money in the center of the table was more than I was used to seeing after working a forty-hour week. Needless to say, I completed the task and left Arizona with $1,600. I paid two months of rent and balled out in IKEA with the rest. I had a brand-new bed. How or why would I deal with anyone who wouldn't make my life simpler? Easier? My body and presence were a form of currency, and I decided to cash in.

Throughout my twenties, these transactional relationships continued. It became easier and easier for me to ask for exactly what I needed while accepting that these surface relationships only existed because we both needed something from one another. I needed and required financial assistance in exchange for their simple need to enter the depths of my pussy, which their thick wallets allowed easy access to. I only asked for the things I absolutely needed. I wasn't asking for shoes or handbags. I would be damned if I was wearing a pair of shoes or a bag that cost more than what was in my bank account. I was on my own. While I never solely depended on men because I always had a job, it sure as hell made it a lot easier for me. These relationships seemed equally balanced at the time. And not one partner was like the next.

I hate to think that you came here for advice on how and where to meet men with money. I don't have any. There literally is no blueprint for this unless you are willing to place yourself on one of those escort websites. I know there's content about going to certain hotel lobby bars or fine dining restaurants and sitting alone, but that has never worked for me. This chapter narrates the mindset of a twentysomething trying to navigate adulthood the best way she knew how. In hindsight, I wish there had been another way. In therapy, this is where I feel the most shame about myself. The depths to which I went to pay rent or simply eat at certain restaurants mortifies me.

I don't want to label these men as sugar daddies because they were more than that to me. I'll refer to them as my "lovers." I met one of them while I was a bartender at an Applebee's. He came in and sat at my bar. His total check was $40, and he added a $40 tip. This caught my attention, and we exchanged contacts with the hope he would become a regular customer at my bar and nothing more. This particular lover was a politician and, though not a millionaire at the time, he could show up in ways that helped me drastically. He made me a ghost employee at his company, and I received a weekly $400 check deposited into my account. I saw him maybe once every two or three months, and whenever we would hang out, it was a fuckin' blast!

Another lover of mine lived in Nigeria. I met him through a friend who posted me on her Instagram page as a #WCW back when Woman Crush Wednesday was a thing. He requested an introduction, and once we got on a call, he immediately sent me $1,000 to show me he wasn't playing. He invited me to Dubai. This was right before I decided to return to school and leave the nightlife. I was ready for a career and didn't want to be a bartender anymore. This man just wanted conversation and sex, and I found it odd that he never wanted oral sex, just missionary. I only saw him twice and got over $30,000 from him.

I had athletes, industry execs, and even a diplomat of a foreign country on my roster. Each of these men showed up in his own way. Whether it was a couple hundred dollars or a couple thousand, it became another source of income. They would cover my travel and bills and eventually help get me through college.

I didn't come from money. We were always just one emergency away from being set back, and I didn't have anyone else to depend on. I couldn't just call Daddy for money. Hell, once I became an adult, he felt entitled and believed we owed him money since he'd paid child support for all those years. GO FUCKIN' FIGURE! I did not have the skills to cook, didn't want children, and got extremely comfortable just being the "fun girl." I wanted to be successful, and I sought financial independence.

Because of these things, I placed being in a REAL relationship in the back of my mind. Unless I met a man with money who could fully provide for me, I had to keep my lovers on standby for a rainy day. I didn't want to cheat. I also didn't know how to effectively communicate to a guy I freely liked that I would need to see these other men to keep my bills paid. So it simply became my usual way of engaging with men. It kept both parties honest for the most part, and everyone got what they wanted. I hadn't seen that take place in any other relationships. My homegirls who were dating men were left in limbo with very few answers as to where they stood. And those who I knew in committed relationships were constantly battling infidelity or financial problems. I felt in control of my emotions and circumstances with these relationships, and they allowed me to ignore my shortcomings as a partner.

The end of my most recent romantic relationship came about when he used my trauma and shame against me in an argument. Through therapy, I discovered that I found it difficult to relive the past decade of my life in which I used my body as a means of survival and validation. This was by far the most harrowing chapter of the book for me to write. I realized my fear of homelessness and my unhealthy relationship with money led me to do whatever I needed to make shit happen. I got comfortable with using my body to barter for currency. Some of these men I didn't find attractive whatsoever, and sex—something that I found enjoyment from—turned into a job. It was not until I started to make my own money and get a firmer grasp on how money was made and spent that I became disgusted by my past actions. Was I really fucking for $1,000, and sometimes even less? And while that is a lot of money for many, I have since reached a place where I buy jeans, a pair of shoes, or a meal and drinks with my homegirls for that same price tag. I had diminished my value to the price of these simple things.

When I'd gotten with my ex, I was six months removed from my corporate career as an accountant at a Big Four firm and was now a full-time entrepreneur. I lived alone in a two-bedroom apartment in the Bronx and had been financially independent for quite some time. Throughout our relationship, he used his narcissistic tactics to silence me. He'd gaslight me and constantly find ways to ruin big moments in my life. Birthdays, professional milestones, and important events were often celebrated in sadness as he would destroy them by starting an argument or breaking up with me. Whenever I questioned him about his change in schedule, attitude, or things he did that violated my boundaries, he would make me feel like I was in the wrong and then punish me with the silent treatment. The silent treatments could last days, weeks, and sometimes even months. And though he had nothing to do with my career, he even began to take credit for my successes while also trying to convince me that it was all temporary.

I told him that I refused to be on that sort of emotional roller coaster anymore, but I also didn't hate him until what would be our final conversation. His weekend availability appeared to shift, and it didn't sit well with me. Men are creatures of habit, and the slightest change to their normal schedule can indicate something's up. I called him to ask if someone else was in the picture. That question set him off. For twenty minutes, he berated me and raised his voice while threatening our relationship yet again. Instead of giving him the power to end us, I ended it. I knew this story all too well. I told him I would be getting off this ride, and I wouldn't allow him to dangle our relationship in my face any longer. I was fed up! I no longer wanted to walk on eggshells, hoping we would remain in this false sense of happiness we had created. I told him it was over and that this wouldn't work. With all the spite in his soul, he wanted me to hurt. How dare I leave him? How dare I question his actions? In the coldest of tones, he uttered:

"Go ahead! Go be single, then. I'm sure you just can't wait to get back to fucking for money."

His words hit me like a ton of bricks. Had this been in the back of his mind during our entire three-year relationship? He'd never even met that version of me. He didn't know THAT girl. I'd opened up to him about what I was working through in therapy, facing my past and the unhealthy relationships I once had with men and sex. The thing in my life that caused so much shame, the secrets I trusted him with, were thrown right back in my face to embarrass me. I was in love with a manipulator. I had fallen hard and allowed a master manipulator to control my psyche. I knew at that moment, however, this would be the last time I would ever speak to him. I could no longer open my legs to him. I could no longer trust this man to protect me. Given all the previous ways in which he'd let me down, there was no fuckin' way I could ever see him the same again.

Sticks and stones may break your bones, but words will never hurt you.

What a fuckin' crock of shit! I was broken. I was depleted. And the reality is, it was because I had not forgiven THAT girl. I still carry so much shame over those decisions. I still haven't found a way to accept the choices I made with many of those men. I have yet to reach the place in this journey where any of it makes complete sense. I may never get to that place while I am still on Earth.

I left that relationship heartbroken and traumatized, but I would be remiss not to mention what truly came from that connection. I found the confidence to believe I was worthy of love and capable of being a phenomenal partner. For the first time, sex took a backseat to intimacy and receiving affection. Even with the opportunity in front of me, no dollar amount would warrant giving myself to someone who is unworthy or doesn't make me feel the way I deserve to feel as a human. I am not an object to be purchased; I am a woman who desires a connection with a person beyond what they offer financially.

With my recent success, money is very different to me now. I look back and can't believe I allowed men to enter me for the price of a tomahawk steak dinner for two. I used to think a man booking me on a flight actually meant something. Now I fly myself around the world and don't bat an eye. The money, the flights, the hotel rooms—none of it meant a goddamn thing. It didn't mean they liked me. It didn't mean they respected me. It was convenient and EASY! This could be a callback to the trauma of going through grade school and not wanting *that word* to be associated anywhere near you. No girl in school wanted the EASY label. Looking back, I feel disgusted by my willingness to be purchased. I feel shame about bartering one of the most precious parts of me in exchange for rent money and trips.

This was the most harrowing chapter for me to write. I saved it for last. It was easier for me to write the chapter about my sexual assault because I was not complicit in that story. In this chapter, I was THAT girl because I chose to be. There are many things we will do along our life journeys that we will find it hard to forgive ourselves for. You may beat yourself up for allowing yourself to be in a situation you know you could have avoided. You may be a prisoner of a traumatic experience that is blocking you from receiving the blessings you deserve. I am still working through the aftermath of having been THAT girl.

I go to therapy, read the kind of books I am writing for you now, and listen to positive-minded growth podcasts. I get up every day and I do the work. I want to share some of the affirmations I tell myself to get past the dark moments to see the brightness of the light ahead of me.

AFFIRMATIONS TO FIND FORGIVENESS

You can repeat these affirmations to yourself.

YOU WOULD NOT BE WHERE YOU ARE TODAY WITHOUT THE OBSTACLES YOU HAVE OVERCOME.

Without the bad, you would not know what good is. The contrast between negative and positive helps us experience the joys of love, connection, gratitude, excitement, and all the other emotions we want to feel. Life is full of contrast: hunger then fullness, waking then sleeping, love and loss, happiness and sadness. It's the contrast that allows us to enjoy the good.

YOU ARE STRONG, RESILIENT, AND A BADASS.

You're reading this book. You're here. Whatever demons you've had to fight did not win! You are a warrior who will face many battles. You never know how strong you are until you have to forgive someone that you'll never receive an apology from.

MY PAST DOES NOT DEFINE ME. I CAN REDEFINE MY STORY STARTING HERE AND NOW.

We have forgiven so many people throughout our lives who have done worse: friends who missed out on important moments, lovers who betrayed our trust, and family members who showed up as strangers in the hardest of times. Forgive yourself the way you have forgiven all these people in your life. You deserve as much grace, if not more, than you've given others.

EVERY NEW DAY IS A CHANCE TO GET IT BETTER.

Look on the bright side. Think of the amazing friends you have, the pet that brings you joy, the job you enjoy working at, or even your most recent vacation. Think of all the amazing things you have in your present. These things may not exist without the path that got you here.

I AM ENOUGH. I AM PERFECT JUST THE WAY I AM. I LOVE MYSELF.

There is nothing more important that you could say, sister!

Patriarchal Bullshit
"If women didn't exist, all the money in the world
would have no meaning."
—Aristotle Onassis (Greek and Argentine
business magnate)[1]

Matriarchal Reply
"Please, do not let fear or laziness be the reason you
continue to struggle financially, I cannot stress this enough."
—Tiffany "The Budgetnista" Aliche
(author of *The One Week Budget: Learn to Create
Your Money Management System in 7 Days or Less!*)[2]

WHY GET PURSES WHEN YOU CAN GET A STOCK PORTFOLIO?

« WEEZYWTF »

I LEARNED ABOUT the hoe hierarchy after discussing my SD (sugar daddy) on *WHOREible Decisions*. Although yes, I am all "YAY FEM-INISM!" on the outside, the patriarchal bullshit has influenced my thought process on sex work. It has influenced our thoughts on almost everything here in the United States, whether we know it or admit it.

If you asked me, being a sugar baby wasn't close to the same thing as being a streetwalker. How could you even compare the two? I thought it was not even comparable to being a regular escort. I mean, they had sex by the hour, and at least I was being treated to lavish dinners first.

My thoughts were simply a product of my naiveté and my environment. I thought of being a sugar baby as the entry point into learning the rules of the housewife life that my mother, my predecessor, taught me. But my dad had "put a ring on it" . . . so, it turned out that being a sugar baby WAS just a glorified way of saying I FUCKED FOR MONEY. Streetwalkers were my sisters in the trade because I was also a sex worker: a bougie-ass one, but a sex worker nonetheless.

I had been on the website Seeking Arrangement from around nineteen to twenty-three years of age. I didn't meet more than probably five men or so, so it wasn't the lifesaver I was expecting it to be. The closest I ever got to landing a big fish was a sexy car auction dealer. We had a nice first meeting, him eyeing me up and down to make sure I was skinny and pretty enough to be his fuck-toy, with me not realizing any of this and just thinking he was decent-looking enough to KISS if I had to.

Like most delusional women on these websites, I was under the impression I would get an allowance of at least 10K per month, shopping sprees, and vacations that I didn't have to have sex on because my SD would just be "enjoying my company."

They all do the same shit, too. Feed you a pipe dream before piping. Tell you how amazing you are, how beautiful, how you're not like the other gold diggers on the site, and how they want to spoil you. Like regular dating, this is all the "boyfriendy type" game.

In the BTP (Boyfriendy Type Person) game, you will experience the following:

- Consistent communication, and maybe even good-morning texts
- Chivalry, compliments, and charm
- Dates, plans made, and promises

And once the pussy is received, the dwindling starts. The calls, the money, the effort, and, in extreme cases, even the cleanliness of his body and home will decline. Alas, pretty similar to regular dating now that I think about it.

Now, if you were an experienced hoe, you would have corrected your course before this even happened. You would realize that you must meet your SD in a more traditional sense. You can't just meet him on a site where you're admitting your thirst for cash.

What's crazy about the effort I put into these sugaring sites is that none paid off as much as the day I went to work at T-Mobile in the Dr. Phillips area of Orlando, Florida. Dr. Phillips is considered a prestigious neighborhood with celebrities who frequent the area, such as Tiger Woods, Shaquille O'Neal, and various members of NSYNC. I never thought I would meet the man who would change my life forever; for the sake of anonymity, let's call him Mark.

Mark (who was way too rich to have T-Mobile, tbh) walked into my store during the fall of 2015. I was twenty-four years old and assistant manager of a company I thought I would be part of forever. He brought one of his kids in for a phone case. I flirted a little, joked a bit, and became part of his morning routine when he grabbed coffee next door. He'd always wave at me and pop in to say a bunch of nothing, and I'd turn on the charm. I knew he was rich as fuck. Beyond the watch and the multiple cars, he just SMELLED like money.

Things changed about a week after one of his daughters broke her phone. They came in to replace it, and when I offered her a case so that she wouldn't break it again, she replied hastily, "My daddy will just buy me another one."

I was in shock. Now, my dad took care of the family, too, but damn . . . Was this some white girl privilege shit? Was it just "I'm rich, you're not" commentary?

So I told Mark, "Well, I need a daddy to buy me whatever I want, too!"

He looked at me very sternly, almost as if he were mad at me, and told me to meet him after work at Ruth's Chris by 8:30 p.m.

I was so fucking nervous. The neighborhood rich guy was asking me out on a date. WHERE THE FUCK WAS HE THE LAST FOUR YEARS I HAD BEEN WORKING A SECOND JOB SCROLLING ON SUGAR SITES???

I rushed home after closing at seven and put on the fanciest dress I could find—Forever 21, but a black dress will usually hide the cheapness. I threw on my Aldo rhinestone shoes and red lipstick and drove my shitty Honda over to the famous steak house. After parking nearby so my car didn't embarrass me at the valet, I hurried to be on time for my first date with Mark.

When I walked in, he was sitting at the bar with a business associate. He scanned me up and down, had his colleague confirm that I was a cutie, and ordered me a dry martini. We discussed how funny our interactions had been at the store. He asked if I was single, and after about thirty minutes, he told me he wanted me on a flight to Panama so that I could join him for a business trip. Now, as much as I wanted to say yes, I had JUST gotten promoted, and I couldn't call out!

Fuck it. I called my boss at the time and told him the truth.

"Listen, you can say no, but the rich guy just asked me on a trip tomorrow and I'll be back at work in two days. Can I go???"

My boss sighed deeply, laughed, and said, "Secure our future!"

There I was (no thanks to the sugaring sites), in my first-class seat to go and meet Mr. Rich Guy. I landed in Panama City, Panama, with a hundred dollars to my name—just enough cash to get my nails and toes done before he got out of work. I was super nervous about what was about to happen, but I figured, *Fucking him will be easier than a forty-hour workweek!*

We met up, shared our first kiss, and headed off to dinner. Everywhere we went, I was oddly turned on by the fact that I was way hotter than him, and people knew I was there for the money. As immoral as that sounds, knowing I'm beautiful enough to be paid for it kinda got me off.

It was clear from the constant ass grabs that he wasn't my real daddy, but in this crazy way, I was attracted to the idea of being there for his money. He had asked me previously about my sexual orientation, and at the time, Scissors and I had been sleeping together on and off. Since he knew I was bisexual, he had the grand idea of taking me to a local bar for prostitutes. In Panama, prostitution is legal, and now I finally understand why so many men want to visit.

The beaches were just okay, but the girls were fucking FIRE. Long legs, dark hair, gorgeous tan skin, and just enough English to get their money.

"Leche, papi?"

"Sexo."

He told me I could pick my favorite girl so we could go home and have sex with her, but little did he know, I picked my favorite girl(s) so that I wouldn't have to fuck at all. I brought back two cuties to his place, watched them suck his dick, then lied and said I wasn't ready to be with a man yet, which, to my surprise, he believed!

I became Mr. Rich Guy's favorite wingman. Clubs, trips to Miami, and a twenty-five-minute flight in his private jet to a Tampa strip club made me literally the only person he wanted to be around. I became the ultimate sugar baby.

My job was to remain beautiful, drama-free, fun, sexy, and the life of the party. I was well-spoken enough to be taken to charity functions and ratchet enough when we entered the VIP room at some of his favorite gentlemen's clubs.

While I enjoyed a life of caviar, champagne, and new purses every few weeks, I felt like something was missing. I compared the things that would frustrate Mark to the average man: choosing which car to drive for the day, being annoyed about why his maid didn't take them out to get washed, and one of his new planes not getting the interior finished in time so he had to fly commercial! Ugh. Poor him!

And poor ME. Because I got a taste and knew I wanted to be able to provide this lifestyle for MYSELF.

I would watch him stay awake into the wee hours of the night to monitor the Asian stock markets, stay on the phone with his advisor, and make trade calls, and I finally got the courage to ask him what it turned out I really wanted.

"Mark, will you teach me how to get rich?"

He laughed at me at first. He asked me what it was that I wanted to buy, and I had to reiterate.

"I don't think you understand. I don't want anything but to not want *for* anything. Please, I want you to teach me how to be financially independent."

I think it was the first time he looked at me beyond my four-year-old boobs and crazy personality.

He realized his wingman was smart enough to have a seat at the table. After that night, he even changed his tone with me. It went from baby goo-goo-ga-ga to him treating me like an adult. He taught me which stocks were most important, why the election would affect the economy, and how to invest in a money manager.

He gave me an initial investment of what I remember to be $10,000, told me to study and decide where to allocate it, and if I made it grow by 15 to 20 percent in a quarter, he would give me another 10K.

I made my investments grow by 35 percent.

I had the willingness to learn and the capability to do more. I started to look at my expenses and saw that I wasn't progressing quickly enough. I needed a challenge and the space for growth, and Orlando wasn't going to give it to me. As much as I knew that I needed that extra cash he was giving me, taking money from a rich man wasn't enough because I wanted to BE a rich man.

My envy of his life inspired me to make a lateral company move to New York City. The day I told him I wanted to leave Florida, he was shocked. He had a million questions and told me to meet him back at the steak house where we'd had our first date.

He looked at me with these puppy dog eyes and said, "Honey, where do you think you're gonna live?"

"I dunno, somewhere in Manhattan probably," I replied.

His face filled with worry as he said, "That must mean Harlem."

I hated how he reeked of white privilege sometimes, but I let it go. After another round of drinks, he said, "All right. I'll get you an apartment. We can get a two-bedroom and be roommates."

He told me exactly what his big three were for the deal to happen:

Two bedrooms and two bathrooms

A doorman and 24/7 concierge

Walking distance to Central Park and Broadway

I couldn't fuckin' believe it. I WAS GOING TO HAVE A LUXURY FUCKING APARTMENT IN NEW YORK CITY!

I got on my shitty laptop the second I got home and found apartments with prices that terrified me. Ain't a concierge the same shit as a doorman? Whatever . . . Anyway, I finally landed on the most beautiful apartment I had ever seen.

The Marc. 260 West 54th Street. It was a full-service building with floor-to-ceiling views, exactly what he wanted. The price tag was $72,000 for the year, and I thought, *He's not going to go for this. Or would he?*

Well, he did. I remember the day the lease finally landed in his assistant's inbox. I was so scared; I felt like he was going to hold this over my head to control me. I was worried he would stalk me and I wouldn't have any freedom.

I had to call the whole thing off. After this realization, I picked up my cell and told him it was too much to ask for and that I didn't think it was right. What he said to me after was so memorable and impactful to the way I viewed money forever.

"Honey, number one, this is not my first rodeo. Number two, I make $50,000 a day. I don't need you to save me money."

Today, as I tell you this story, I am ashamed to say I felt like I shouldn't have taken this man's money. WHY THE HELL DID I CARE? He was rich, and I was a month behind on my credit card bill. What I learned was that I was counting his pockets with the same eyes I had for mine. At that point, I was making 75K a year—a lot for a twenty-year-old, but my salary was thirty-five hours of work for him. The man was a multi-MILLIONAIRE.

So I was moving to the Big Apple with no rent and a sugar daddy to take care of me. I also had all the proper financial practices going for me. I allocated what my average rent would have been at the time to a savings account, boosted my 401(k), had the max taxes taken out of my checks, gave my parents some extra spending money, and continued to milk my SD for stock advice.

He only visited twice a year; during those two trips, he bought me about $10K to $15K's worth of clothes and bags. I returned all of them, since he always paid in cash, and kept stacking my money. I remember the last time I saw him; he didn't say he wouldn't renew the lease, but it felt kinda final. We went to Sapphire, a strip club near the apartment. Per usual, he handed me cash; I pocketed half and gave the rest to the girls. On the walk home, I knew I was going to fuck him that night.

We got home and I gave myself a hoe bath to hurry up and make sure he didn't fall asleep. He was lying in bed as he waited for the Asian markets to pop up on the screen when I came in wearing my finest lingerie. I had heels, my hair in a perfect ponytail, and the best-scented Bath and Body Works I could find. I wanted to seduce him, thank him, and show him that his money was worth it.

He damn near threw the remote to the wall when he flipped the blanket over and aggressively pulled his short and curved pink dick out while he jerked off to the sight of me. For some reason, I didn't mind that it wasn't big; I didn't mind his stomach or hairy chest. He was actually attractive to me. Or maybe I was just finally playing out this escort fantasy in my head.

I got on my knees and told him to stand up and come to me, following his eyes the entire time he walked over. I started sucking him off with my hands laid perfectly on my knees (as my Dom had taught me in the apartment Mark paid for). It was the perfect act of submission and seduction. He kept talking about how amazing my mouth felt, how he felt so special that he got to feel how warm it was. He continued with some unexpected dirty talk about how he was sorry he didn't have a pussy for me, and I started to suck his dick even harder so he would just shut up.

He told me to bend over on the bed; I felt like a condom wasn't coming into this situation, so I just prayed he had no STDs because the good Lord knows I wouldn't have kept this old fuck's baby. He started to pump a little too fast, but it was kinda good! Our chemistry out of the bedroom proved itself once the sex started, and I imagined the entire time that I was a high-end escort who had a client to please.

It wasn't really a fantasy in the end; it was my reality. He came on my face and immediately passed out on the bed. I watched his dick shrivel up before I went to go clean off. I stared at myself in the mirror and thought about how sexy I was. Even though I knew I never cared to do this again, I was so happy that I had.

My SD ended up getting a girlfriend who became very jealous of the "gay bestie" he had in New York City. She made up some whole lie that I contacted her from a fake page and harassed her about my deep feelings for him.

AS IF!!! Why the fuck would I even mess up my own money? But he believed her, and I was off to live alone in the Lower East Side.

When I think back on him, I remember that podcast episode when I learned about the hoe hierarchy. Some women have a choice, and some have a circumstance. I chose to fuck him for money. I didn't have to have a luxury apartment in New York, new clothes, or a stock portfolio. It was ALWAYS in me; I was ALWAYS meant to get ahead. I was born a hustler, and my time would have come. Yet, I was no better than the woman who had to sell her body on the streets to feed herself and be able to afford a bed for the night. We are not above any woman, just because we were born into a "better" family or got a better education. Most of us are a few paychecks away from a different lifestyle. It just so happened that with Mark, I made him my job, so that I could afford the lifestyle of luxury that I desired.

I thought Mark was the privileged one, but considering the circumstances, I must understand that the treatment I received was a privilege in itself. I did what I did to have *more* things, not basic necessities. I was fortunate enough to be in a safe situation where I had a CHOICE as to whether or not I wanted to have sex. Sadly, the cookie doesn't always crumble that way. Many people have put their lives at risk by engaging in the same type of behavior that I did. I want to honor those who did not have a choice and who were forced into these situations, all those people who have been abused or even lost their own lives at the hands of violence from having to be in sex work scenarios.

Looking back on this time also taught me crucial lessons regarding how I would deal with my finances in the future. Knowing how to manage your money is essential for achieving financial stability and INDEPENDENCE. This freedom is what I want for all of us. I want us all to win! Understanding how to handle money reduces stress and helps avoid debt, allowing you to build a secure future. By mastering these skills, you can achieve financial freedom, plan for retirement, and handle unexpected expenses with confidence and peace of mind. Financial literacy empowers you to be informed.

On that note, I will end with a few of the best books and podcasts that can help you learn to manage your cash:

BOOKS

- *Get Good with Money: Ten Simple Steps to Becoming Financially Whole* by Tiffany Aliche
- *We Should All Be Millionaires: A Woman's Guide to Earning More, Building Wealth, and Gaining Economic Power* by Rachel Rodgers
- *Financial Feminist: Overcome the Patriarchy's Bullsh*t to Master Your Money and Build a Life You Love* by Tori Dunlap

PODCASTS

- *That Moment* with Daymond John
- *Brown Ambition* with Mandi Woodruff and Tiffany Aliche
- *Earn Your Leisure* with Rashad Bilal and Troy Millings (This show is actually taped at my production studio locations between LA and NYC; talk about a return on my investment!)

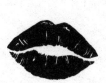

Patriarchal Bullshit
"As time passes, the joy of the victory fades, just like a wife becomes old and loses her charm."
—Sriprakash Jaiswal (Indian union coal minister)[1]

Matriarchal Reply
"Why would a man need both a wife and a mistress? A smart man would seek out and fall in love with a woman who can play both."
—Brenda Jackson (quoted from *Delaney's Desert Sheikh*)[2]

DO MARRIED MEN REALLY TREAT YOU BETTER?

« MANDII B »

I WOULD LIKE to let it be known that I have been a proud member of the Side Chick Committee, on the board of the Mistress Missions, and an elected official to the Jezebel Justice League. Does that make me a piece of shit? Perhaps.

"Ignorance is bliss, 'tis folly to be wise." Not knowing something can be more comfortable than knowing it. I thought I was secure in knowing I existed in a man's life among many other women. I didn't mind sharing him willingly and signed up to be a side piece because at least he was being "honest" with me. The lack of intimacy, affection, and even conversation with a man didn't bother me because I had never seen or experienced anything else. Many of my relationships struggled to breach the surface, and I liked it that way, without diving deep into who he truly was. I always saw things as black-and-white; I never got lost in the gray or delusion in my relationships (or so I thought). It wasn't until I fell for someone and experienced the magic that comes with love, intimacy, and care that I felt shame about how I'd allowed myself to exist with so many men from my past. That's the funny thing about dating and navigating life. It's hard to miss something you've never had. But boy, it becomes the standard once you experience something so amazing.

Now I am pretty certain that this particular chapter is going to piss quite a few of you off, if I haven't already. I get it. I get it. No woman respects another woman who actively pursues a relationship with a man who is already "taken." From grade school, we are taught to view relationships only as a duo when we pass notes between classes and are asked to be someone's valentine with a card featuring a pop band and a cheesy phrase. Once you are someone's boyfriend or girlfriend, there are rules around behaving or interacting with anyone who wasn't stamped as "yours." As we get older, with monogamy in the forefront and marriage as the end goal for most, one thing is certain: you can only have one partner. This is odd when you consider that "only 17 percent of human cultures are strictly monogamous," according to an article on monogamy and human evolution in the *New York Times*. "The vast majority of human societies embrace a mix of marriage types, with some people practicing monogamy and others polygamy."[3] But I was taught that if you were in a relationship and chose to step out on your partner, you were a cheating adulterer. If you were a woman who decided to engage with a person who was already in a relationship with another woman, you were a homewrecking piece of shit.

As women, we were automatically indoctrinated into a society with another set of rules—the Girl Code. You know some of the unspoken **Girl Code Rules**, right?

- Never date your friend's ex.
- Never crush on your friend's crush.
- Don't post photos online unless both of you look good.
- Keep secrets a secret and don't share with anyone unless given direct permission.
- If you see your friend's boyfriend cheating, TELL HER!

But what loyalty do I have to a woman that I don't even know? Somehow, those rules were included under the umbrella of "treat others how you'd want to be treated." Somehow, you'd be ostracized and kicked out of being a Girl's Girl if you broke any of these rules, even with a stranger. Hell, I didn't make any vows to be honest and trustworthy and hold someone down through sickness and health. I want to take you through the mindset of a side chick, and when I felt comfortable and even proud to wear that title . . . but bear with me, because I will also get to the part where I hold my own selfish ass accountable for being so damn naive.

You may be surprised to learn that 70 percent of all Americans engage in some form of infidelity in their lives. In the United States, 20 to 25 percent of heterosexual married women and 20 to 40 percent of heterosexual married men will have an affair.[*] It's pretty wild that we can't just assume that a person hitting on us is actually available to us.

In my twenties, I did not care what a man had going on when he wasn't with me. He could be a whole God-fearing man, married to his high school sweetheart, and Father of the Year and I wouldn't give a damn. If I wanted him, I got him. If he wanted me, his relationship status meant little to nothing. As long as I was getting what I wanted out of the ordeal, then what did it matter?

I will break down some psychological thoughts of a side chick to help you understand a bit more:

GUILT FREE—Often, it begins innocently. It could start with a lie from the other party about their relationship status, or sometimes a woman just doesn't give a damn. Either way, they remove their role in hurting the other woman and place that responsibility on the man.

CRAVING—Being a side chick thrills her now. She enjoys the dopamine of being strongly desired and sought after by her lover. The idea that this man is risking it all for her keeps her engaged.

REASONING—There's comfort in finally being "chosen" or desired in this way by a man, and the relationship seems to work in many instances. While some side chicks can be heartless and lean into the monetary advantages that can come from this sort of arrangement, it's hard for many not to catch feelings. Then denial sets in, and the inevitable emotions come up.

EMOTIONS—This is where comfort and denial collide, creating a beautiful balance of hope. The side chick may begin to compare his love for her to his love for his partner. There's also a shift to her wanting to be The Main, The Primary, and #1 in his life. This could happen early in the relationship or take time, but best believe it will probably happen.

REALITY HITS—The side chick has to decide whether they will seek to destroy the relationship of her lover OR finally find self-worth and choose to leave this relationship. Unfortunately, more often than not, the emotions are so high that the side chick fears losing this person altogether, and everything tends to get complicated.

Now, what were the things I wanted? All-expense-paid trips, lavish dinners, and money, of course. Was I trying to bear children for a man? No. Did I have my fairy-tale wedding planned out in my head? Nah. Did I want to diminish my own existence to simply serve a man? Fuck no! I wanted all of the best parts of a man without any of the responsibility. I didn't picture myself having a man's dinner cooked for him when he got off from a long workday. I didn't feel mentally ready to be there for a man during his highs and lows. I simply didn't want the full responsibility of being "wifey." I wanted just the best parts of a man: the laughs, the fun, the money, and the dick!

Besides the material elements of these relationships, I also received the best versions of these men while also being allowed to be myself. I wasn't watching the things I said or shapeshifting myself to be what I thought a man would want in a wife. I got to be the homie, the lover, the friend. I got to be extremely honest with them and receive the same in return. Why would he have to lie to me? Lying is a part of human communication, and more often than not, a lie within a partnership is told to (a) preserve the relationship, (b) spare feelings, or (c) not be held accountable for their own behavior. It was a win for me to feel like I beat the game of dating by landing a man who could be honest and transparent with me because, let's be serious here, (a) I wasn't in a relationship worth preserving, (b) our feelings for one another had a ceiling, and (c) how the fuck do you have the authority to really hold someone else's husband or partner accountable?

DO MARRIED MEN REALLY TREAT YOU BETTER? Let me explain where this chapter title came from. In many ways, they often do treat you better than single men. Married men will frequently shower you with lavish gifts, keep interactions light, and rarely question you about what you're doing when they're not around. The secrets, lies, and bullshit that often come with meeting single men who are actively dating and entertaining multiple women normally don't apply. Married men will also show up better with their mistresses than they do with their own wives. As I mentioned, you get a different, more fun version of the man when the stresses of life's responsibilities aren't added to the relationship.

I've been a part of some of the most triflin'-ass scenarios, too. While I have never slept in the bed that a man shared with his wife, when I look back at it, I probably partook in some pretty scandalous acts. I remember one of my ex-lovers inviting me to his preseason game. He was a married NFL player, and we had been friends long before we started fuckin'. Years later, during a trip to New York, we blurred the lines and became friends with benefits. There was never a conversation about what this meant to our relationship, but we fell into being lovers.

When he invited me to the game, there weren't many details except for the fact that he would also be bringing his friends from back home. I had met quite a few of his friends up to this point, so it didn't bother me; however, he didn't tell me how I was a part of his whole mischievous, toxic-ass plans! He sent me my first-class ticket and the name of the hotel I would stay at. Because I flew in on game day and he would already be at the stadium by the time I landed, he had his closest friend pick me up from the airport, bring me to the hotel to change, and come to the game with me. The weather was extremely shitty that day. It was raining on and off and the sky was dark gray. Because of the weather, he let me know I'd be in a suite to keep me dry. He was texting me throughout the morning, making sure I was good, and told me to stay with his friends until after the game.

I had purchased a shirt at the airport that morning to come dressed to root for the home team. In my bedazzled NFL tank and ripped jeans, I walked into the suite, and to my surprise, his wife and children were right there. No, this motherfucker did not fly me here to be in a suite with his fucking wife and kids!!! I kept my cool and stayed close to his friends. I found a beer, made a plate of nachos, and conducted myself accordingly, which meant that I put my feelings in check and considered his situation over my own emotions. It would have been entirely catastrophic to make a scene. He brought his friends as decoys and made it look like I was there as a guest of one of his boys. I peeped the game. Play on.

Following the game, I questioned why he would put me in a suite with his wife. He innocently responded that he didn't want me sitting out in the rain for the game. That answer sufficed, and like the good girl I was, I made sure to let him know that I played my cool and stuck close to his boys. I remember questioning how he would get away with being with me that evening. Whew! The self-ishness jumped out. I didn't think much about how distraught the wife would be to know I was actually there for her husband. I knew that they hadn't agreed on an ethical non-monogamous relation-ship. At the time, however, I didn't know the heartache that came with cheating and betrayal. He brought me in and would end the evening with me. The practice facility happened to be over an hour away from where they lived, and he used the excuse of staying close to the facility to get more sleep the morning after their win. He was actually staying right downtown with me, in the room he got me, so that I could suck his soul out in congratulatory fashion.

It's safe to say that playing this role for as long as I did, with the many men I did, sullied my desire to be a wife or #1. I was never jealous of their position in a man's life. Here they were, being lied to, cheated on, and completely unaware that their husband likes to hold his legs up and get his ass eaten. She's home taking care of the kids while I'm jumping off the back of a yacht in the Caribbean, trying the freshest of ceviches, and taking back tequila shots. She has to deal with his mood swings and his snoring every night and cater to his every need while I get the fun version of him for a few days.

I do not want to make it seem like being a side chick is all bells and whistles. The reality is, as a side chick, you don't get many of the perks of actually being with a person. Most holidays you spend alone; you get used to celebrating either the day before or the day after. You aren't around or as heavily involved with their family. You may know all the friends, but you won't have that relationship with his mom or kids. Reality will sink in over time, that this whole thing may not be "real." I remember not hearing from one of my partners for two days, only to find out he'd ended up in the hospital. I spiraled, thinking about the reality that no one would notify me if he were terminal or dying. I wouldn't be able to visit him in the hospital. Would I even be able to attend his funeral? Could I be there without shame? Here I was, giving my all to a man I wouldn't even be able to grieve publicly. How is that not embarrassing?

The side chick narrative worked for me for years until I ended up in the other seat. My three-year relationship with the person I believed to be my soulmate had finally ended. Three weeks after truly walking away I was met with another nail in the coffin of that relationship and a twist of the dagger to my heart. A woman contacted me on Instagram with information about my previous partner. We exchanged numbers, and early in the morning, I received information that truly devastated me. Was I surprised by what I learned? Not quite. But was I hurt? Absolutely. She was one of four women he was cheating on me with. He had been with her on that trip he took to Panama for suits, when he said that he wanted to spend more solo time together and stay out of the sex club. The night he claimed he left his cell phone in the taxicab and couldn't contact me for hours, he had just left her house. They knew about my relationship with him; I was the only one in the dark. Did he love me more because he chose to lie to me to preserve our relationship? Did he lie to me to shield my feelings? Fuck all that bullshit. He fuckin' embarrassed me!

Just a month after this call, I had another woman-to-woman experience when one of the other women saw me eating outside a Mexican restaurant in Brooklyn. She chose to come to me and share what her relationship had been with my ex. She sat in my face and spewed the same bullshit I had once believed. This lady had the nerve to place her six-month relationship with him over my three-year relationship simply because she felt he was honest with her the entire time and lied to me. I was stung. Karma came and knocked me fucking dead in my tracks. My previous ignorance confronted me. We ended the conversation with me buying us a round of tequila shots. I couldn't do anything but accept that I had once been this person. I was once the person who would cause this type of hurt and betrayal in another relationship.

So let's bring it back to this chapter's title once again. **DO MARRIED MEN REALLY TREAT YOU BETTER?** In hindsight, that entire mindset was nothing more than a facade constructed by a naive individual who still had a lot to learn about themselves. While I was benefiting in some ways, I realized that I was being used as a pawn in someone else's story, and the role was so insignificant that I wouldn't even be nominated for an Oscar in a supporting role. The power you think you hold in that relationship dwindles to nothing once that person decides you no longer serve a purpose. This can happen when they end their primary relationship and don't choose you as the replacement, or they find another woman with just as few—or even fewer—requirements.

It wasn't until I felt true love and heartbreak that I could grow out of my selfishness. Experiencing love and finding self-esteem allowed me to realize I was so comfortable being number two because I lacked morals and self-worth, and allowed myself to be an easy target for men seeking a woman who would accept the bare minimum. When accepting the role of number two, you are okay with taking the crumbs from a person. You may convince yourself you have enough to be fulfilled if you gather enough crumbs. Don't lie to yourself. You deserve the whole damn cake!

20 THINGS TO BUILD YOURSELF UP

1. **RECITE AFFIRMATIONS**—They are cheesy until they aren't . . .
2. **TAKE AN EXERCISE CLASS**—Try something new
3. **GO FOR A WALK**—Get outside and get moving
4. **WEAR BEAUTIFUL UNDERWEAR**—For no one but yourself
5. **READ AN UPLIFTING SELF-HELP BOOK**—Some of my favorites are
   - *What I Know for Sure* by Oprah Winfrey
   - *Set Boundaries, Find Peace* by Nedra Glover Tawwab
   - *The Four Agreements* by Don Miguel Ruiz
   - *The Let Them Theory* by Mel Robbins
6. **JOURNAL**—So you know where your head is at
7. **MEDITATE**—Quiet your mind
8. **TAKE CREDIT**—Brag about the good things you do
9. **GET YOUR HAIR DONE**—When you know you look good, you feel good

10. CONNECT TO THE PEOPLE YOU LOVE—Text, call, Zoom, plan a dinner

11. TAKE A SOLO TRIP—You know how it worked out for me ;-)

12. TAKE YOURSELF OUT TO DO SOMETHING YOU LOVE—Dinner, a movie, a museum, a concert

13. HELP SOMEONE ELSE—Volunteer, or buy flowers for someone who needs a pick-me-up

14. SMILE—Simply smiling lifts your spirits

15. LAUGH—Is seriously the best medicine

16. GET THERAPY—Be the person in your family to slay that generational trauma

17. REFRESH YOUR SPACE—Remove the clutter around you to declutter your mind

18. REST—Deep rest is necessary to recharge

19. ENJOY HEALTHY FOOD—You are what you eat

20. KNOW YOUR WORTH—You deserve to be treated like royalty. We all do.

Patriarchal Bullshit
"All women are born evil.
Some just realize their potential
later in life than others."
—Jean Giraudoux (French author, essayist, diplomat)[1]

Matriarchal Reply
"Fall in love with yourself, with life,
and then with whoever you want."
—Frida Kahlo (Mexican painter)[2]

DOES LOVE
SHOW UP WHEN YOU
AREN'T LOOKING?*

« WEEZYWTF »

I have thought long and hard about whether
I should include the current part of my life in this book.
SPOILER ALERT, Y'ALL: Ya girl found LOVE!

Here are my anxious thoughts:
OMG what if we break up?
What if this book gets published and it doesn't work out?
Here is the fucking reality:
WHO. CARES.

I have felt so much liberation and freedom from the stories that you have read, but I would be a liar if I said that love hasn't been my goal in dating. Along the way, I have had some amazing experiences—enough to make a popular podcast. But my intention when approaching dating has always been a fairy-tale ending. I know it's possible because I grew up with two parents who are still madly in love today!

Yet, I have been so heartbroken by my previous relationships that the confidence I carry in everyday life was challenging to carry in love. The thing that attracted men to me, my confidence, was the very thing that dwindled once they had me. I was so familiar with pain that love felt like reaching for a flame. I expected it to hurt. How could I trust that I would be enough?

Although it's cliché as a muthafucka, I didn't become enough until I really fell in love with myself first. I started my single years swiping every guy, hoping they would be my husband, to just swiping for fun. Going outside in amazing outfits, not just "in case I met the one" but because I WANT TO FEEL SEXY. After spending fourteen years (between sixteen and twenty-nine) with the male gaze in mind, my people-pleasing days were finally over, and I know that's precisely why I met him. Timing is everything; I couldn't have had a love like this in 2018 because I was still healing. I just didn't know it.

We were right for each other the day we met, and that is why I can write this chapter for you today. This wasn't a story that I had planned to put in this book because it had yet to happen. But now that it has happened and I am in love, I can't think of a better way to discuss my progression.

I'm not going to go as far as to say I was thirsty, but I was confused about why love wasn't happening for me. I've never been a patient person. Maybe it's just the way I'm built, but if I want it, I NEED IT NOW.

That *now* mentality led me to make a lot of mistakes. When I thought about love before, I thought about partnership and how well someone would fit into my life. As long as they looked how I wanted them to and were good on paper, I figured, "HE'S THE ONE!" I never listened to what men were actually saying to me. I never thought about if they respected me—as I've proven in more than one chapter at this point. #O1Bae

I'd never considered what real compatibility would look like in my romantic relationships. In friendships, it's easy to have a friend who's the opposite of you. You don't need to build a life, have kids, and share a house and a bank account with all your friends. Compatibility can be minimal.

I'd never sat down with myself and asked what I now believe are vital questions for a prosperous and sustainable relationship. When I did, this is what the questions looked like:

1. Do I love the way this person sees the world?
2. Do we find pleasure in the same activities, and if we don't, can we support each other?
3. Do we share the same values and have the same overall moral compass?
4. Can we make each other feel safe and heard during disagreements?
5. Are we able to honor each other's needs EASILY?
6. Is the sex bomb?

Before my love growth spurt, number six was all that I looked for.

I remember my first love. We were so crazy about each other that we got matching tattoos and wrote each other love notes at work. My second love was the guy who pledged himself to me under the moonlight and said he would die without me by his side . . . Lies.

Then there was the love that was a surface love—maybe we should just call it *like*. You don't NEED them, but you don't want anyone else for now. Realistically, you know something better will come along. And when it does, you will leave.

I had felt love before, and I felt like a junkie always trying to chase that first high. I remember walking around New York, hoping and praying that I would meet "him" when I turned the next corner. That's what movies made falling in love seem like. I would be lying underneath a tree in Central Park with a novel in my hand when the soccer ball he was kicking landed on me.

"Oh shit! Are you okay?" he would say frantically.

I'd be mad, but once the sun shone on his face and I got a glimpse of how hot he was, I'd say coyly, "Yeah, I guess I'm all right."

I'd hand him the ball, and when he helped me up, I'd fall into his arms, and a bitch turns into your modern-day Cinderella who gets saved. I'm not sure what he's supposed to be saving me from. He's the dumbass who kicked a ball at me in the first place.

Of course, that didn't happen because life is not a movie. The way my unorthodox life works, there was no place for me to meet the person of my dreams other than on a fuckin' dating app. Oh, how I despise the fact that at my wedding one day, I'll have to admit to everyone that my hoe ass was swiping for new dick when, instead, I found my life partner.

One weekday in July, I was aimlessly cruising Hinge when I saw his profile. There were photos of him in front of a Basquiat exhibit. There he was, beautiful, tatted, with luscious dreadlocks. He was standing in front of one of the pieces I happened to have inked on my arm. But I was tired of looking for yet another SIGN that someone was meant to be with me, and I was meant to be with them. He was sexy, and I needed a new dude to fuck in New York. Since

I bounce between coasts, I figured I'd get my roster up until I met "THE ONE."

The interesting thing about timing in relationships is that just because you are ready for one thing doesn't necessarily mean the other person is in the same space. I'd had so many men tell me they weren't prepared for a relationship. I would sob in confusion while looking up at my ceiling and screaming, "Why isn't it ME?!?" before crying myself to sleep.

I'd had year after year of seeing men I've loved end up with someone else, wondering why I wasn't the one they had chosen. Spending hours going through their new beau's profile, thinking it was because she was skinnier than me, prettier, thicker, maybe funnier than I was. I'd send her profile to my friends so they could also validate my feelings while I'd berate another woman just to make myself feel better. I'd go into full-on stalker mode to figure out exactly how, why, and when I would become worthy of love like them. Why couldn't I have been chosen, too? But it all makes sense today because my time for love wasn't until now.

When this love came to me, I was completely ready to receive it. And so was he. This was the key. Once we started talking about our lives, it was clear there was no way that we should not have met before we did.

With every conversation, we realized how much we had in common. We would ask each other, "How in the hell is it possible that we haven't met before?" We went to the same sex clubs, concerts, museums, parks, and travel spots. Where had he been?

I hope the answer will inspire anyone who isn't happy and does not want to be single.

He wasn't ready for ME. And I wasn't prepared for HIM, either. We were not in spaces where it would have worked before NOW.

You haven't met your person yet because they aren't ready to be the fully formed partner that you need. Yes, that person. exists for you, but maybe they are still learning to fix those things that make you feel the ick. And you're still developing as well.

Maybe you're the type of person who overthinks everything; perhaps you're overly emotional, and you are learning how to manage that so as not to drive your future partner away. Maybe you love to be listened to, and your person is right in the middle of learning to be a better communicator.

In my case, he wasn't ready to be my man in the summer of 2022 when I was out here looking for love. How could he? He had to get over his ex, and to do that, he had to have his hoe years. He needed time to grow and mature.

How could I have been his girl? Besides the fact that we didn't know each other yet, I needed those last few months of therapy before we met to stop harboring resentment toward men in general. My need for speed would have driven him insane had I not learned that patience is a virtue through meditation and spiritual books.

A few years before I met him, one of my girlfriends, Rasheeda, said something impactful. "Baby, why are you rushing? This could be your LAST summer single. Enjoy yourself! Who told you you need to move faster than you already are?"

And it hit me: we have been trained to rush a process that, frankly, the patriarchy has forced upon us.

Maaaan (literally), why can't women just have sex, get the fuck off, and enjoy some pleasure in the meantime? Why must we treat our lives like a giant round of speed dating? *It. Will. Come.* And when it does, you'll understand precisely what I mean about this next phase of my life.

Before it came, the frivolous sex was a story to write home about.

Shit, it's how I made a living with the podcast. The hot guy I went on a few dates with then finally fucked the shit out of after a New York summer night. The wild three-way make out I had with two girls after snorting lines at the Soho Grand. The third date who I let fondle me in the back of an Uber before we got upstairs and had no-frills sex until dawn.

But does anything top sex when you're in LOVE? This is a serious question.

The sex where love takes over. The space beyond lust. Instead of just looking at how sexy someone is, you find yourself needing to tell them they're beautiful instead, and you don't just mean physically. Sexy alone just doesn't mean enough anymore.

It's a little bit crazy how love can make your brain forget everything you said you'd never do.

"I'll never get peed on."

"I'll never let you taste my blood."

"I'll never let you fuck another woman."

I'm not saying I did those things . . . Okay, maybe I did, but who cares? Love is fuckin' nutty! And speaking of nut, is that when I started to feel love? When he began nutting in my pussy?

What does it mean when your body starts to crave someone? When your physical existence needs to be bound somehow with the person you love?

I know we all have heard the "CUM FOR ME, DADDY. PUT IT DEEP IN ME" lines. You know, the stuff we learn in porn. But what about when love strikes? Has your body ever been so in tune with another person that you literally were obsessed with their orgasm?

I remember the day I thought I would die without it. Thanksgiving Eve, but there was nothing particularly special about the day.

Maybe it was the full moon. Maybe the tequila. But it was the day that I could feel my pussy craving his release. Insanely. I remember staring into his eyes as if I needed to confirm his orgasm was real. I desperately needed to feel the throbbing sensation, his warmth filling up inside of me. I told him that my body was made for him, that I was his. That I was BORN for him to cum inside of me. I was obsessed with feeling his orgasm because I wanted a part of him inside of me. Forever.

Am I not . . . CRAZY?!

Anyway, just don't have sex as a Pisces on a full moon.

Love is the feeling I get when I hear him buzz my apartment; sometimes, I feel like I'm gonna pee my pants because I'm so fucking excited to see him! (Not like the time he peed on me in Tulum in that Jacuzzi tub where people had full view of us from the street. But you know, the kind of pee when you're super anxious.)

Love is the feeling he had when he watched *Saltburn* without me. When that infamous scene came on, where the guy fingered that girl on her period and rubbed it all over her chest and on his face, he texted me, "Tell me when you see IT." I didn't know what IT was until IT came on the screen. He told me, "I would fucking do that with you."

Love is the feeling we got in the middle of a foursome with two lesbians in Sayulita, Mexico. I was wrist-deep in some Midwestern girl's pussy when I saw him smirking at me. He loved watching me enjoy myself. We were gazing at each other while inside of two other people, so enthralled with our own sexual energy that we couldn't tell that the other couple was on the brink of their own breakup. When we left the girls' apartment, they were arguing so loud we could hear it from the street. "WELL, IF YOU WANTED TO BE WITH A MAN JUST FUCKING BE WITH ONE!!!" I couldn't believe it—the engaged duo who'd approached US for sex couldn't get it together! (Meanwhile, we were professing our love for each other and how safe we felt and started planning our next vacation.)

The lust and love combination epitomizes what we're all looking for. The moment you look at someone and you know how badly you want to kiss them, make love to them, but goddamn, at the same time you're thinkin', *I love how your brain works. I love everything about you.*

I remember the night he told me what I had already been feeling for a few weeks. (But I damn sure wasn't going to say it first.) We were on vacation. He was inside of me. And this was the first time anyone had ever said it then.

I remember exactly how he said it . . .

Him: I love your pussy.

More sex.

Him: Do you know how much I love your body?

More sex.

Him: I love your big ol' butt.

More sex.

Him: I fucking love the way you . . .

More sex. He looks at me intensely.

Him: I LOVE YOU.

Looking at me like he really sees me. All of me.

Him: I LOVE YOU! DO YOU HEAR ME?
Me: Mmmm, yeahhh. I love you, too.

On the inside, I was GUSHING!!! *AHHHH!!! GOT HIS ASS!!!*
I felt so ecstatic and happy—he loved me! After he came, I
rushed to the bathroom. It was in part to pee out the cum because
I mean, *hello*, no urinary tract infections over here! But it was also
the only way to immediately text in my favorite group chat with my
friends, Andre and Asante.

Me: OMG. HE SAID HE LOVES ME, YALL! Just fuckin'
now during sex, omgongoh ahhhhh!
Andre: WHOAAA.
Asante: Damn, he said it IN THE PUSSY THO????
Me: So!?!? Does that mean he doesn't mean it??
Andre: I mean . . . I don't know.

I was crushed. Was this what they did? Did guys just say they
love you during sex?
I could barely sleep. Shit! Why the fuck did I text these bozos?
They didn't get it! UGH! Or did they? My thoughts kept me up
until 7 a.m., and I dragged myself to the pool with a little attitude in
fear that my "I love you" was just said on a whim.
We had a few drinks, and I forgot about the whole debacle. After
a swim, I got out. He spanked my ass and told me how cute my lil'
butt was.

I said, "Lil'? I thought you said I have a big butt?"

He started laughing and said, "That's just sex talk, baby."

My face turned red with rage as I got up from my seat and said, "Oh, so you just say shit you don't mean during sex, then?"

He grabbed me by my towel and said, "Oh, you talkin' about when I said I love you last night? Nah, because I meant that shit." I immediately felt stupid. "That's what you wanted to bring up? Because I DO LOVE YOU."

I smiled sheepishly and sat back down. HA! The group chat didn't know JACK SHIT!

Now, I love my friends . . . but what I learned from this moment was to stop tellin' 'em every damn thing. Our friends know all of our past fuckups. They're like a database filled with our traumas and the scar tissue we associate with our exes. It's perfectly fine until they remind us of our previous angst because they tell us why we haven't met "THE ONE."

I love the way he loves me. I love the way he notices my energy shift when I put on a dress that doesn't fit the way I like. He tells me how fucking sexy I am before the thought permeates my brain. I love how he can't walk past me without a kiss on my neck, and finds a way to touch, dance, or talk about future plans out of nowhere.

One afternoon, I was frying some fish. I could see him staring at me . . . so, of course, I fixed my posture so I would look perfect to him.

"You are going to be so beautiful pregnant. I can't wait to watch your body change, watch you glow, watch your breasts change, your lips, everything."

I looked back at him and thought, *Does this nigga think I look fat right now? Why the fuck is he thinking about me being pregnant?* But then I realized that when he sees me, he sees his life—his plans, desires, and all the fantasies that accompany them.

I hope he loves me the way I love him, too. He's not a morning person. I am. Sometimes, I miss him so much when he's sleeping. I hope and pray that a fucking bus goes by and hits the horn just so I don't have to spend another hour without him. I sneak out of bed to cook him breakfast so he can wake up and feel special. Serving him feels deeper than sex; it feels like a calling. I love the way we show our love for each other.

After one of our podcast's live shows in New York City at Sony Hall, Mandii and I were on such a crazy high. Fifteen hundred fans screaming our name, lights flashing, and a standing ovation. And all I wanted to do was curl up into a ball with him and go home. He sat in the back of the Uber with me on the way to my after-party. He led me into deep breathing, took my shoes off, rubbed my feet, and told me how proud he was of me. He felt my shift, and not because I had said anything about how stressed I was.

The way we want to share everything is ridiculous—like best friends but worse. One time we went to a music festival in the jungle and lost our friends with the MDMA, so all we were left with was acid. Since I'd met him, he'd always said he'd never do it . . . but somehow, when I let it sit on my tongue, he took some, too—only because, he said, "We always need to be on the same vibration." The comedown was insane, but we laughed fifteen hours later that at least we'd thought we would die of highness together.

I always wondered how my parents stayed so in love over the years. Now I know. The other day, my father, who's in a wheelchair, was struggling to pick something up. My mom watched him from across the room and said, "OH, COME ON! IT'S NOT LIKE YOU'RE HANDICAPPED!" My dad cracked up laughing. She came over to pick it up, he kissed her, and they continued their silly game.

It's that kinda shit. The shit that nobody understands but the two of you.

We laugh constantly in ways that make people think we're fucking crazy. Sometimes, when I return from the bathroom at a restaurant and I'm doing a little sexy walk, he notices how I'm aiming to get everyone's eyes on me. I sit back at our table, and he stares me up and down and says, "YOU FUCKING WHORE. Look at you. You can't help yourself, you slut! You want to fuck everyone in here, don't you?!!"

He tries to hold his lips together, so I don't see his smile as he breaks character, and I burst out in giggles. I know, it's ridiculous, but it's the shit that makes us laugh.

I love when he tells me he's infatuated with me. The word feels excessive, but I know why he uses it. Because his love has no boundaries.

I had just come back from a long work trip in LA, and the day I arrived, my cycle was in full throttle and unexpected. I started to cry in the car on the way back home when he asked me what was wrong. I told him how gross I felt, how I was so sad that I couldn't make love to him the way I wanted because I would make a fucking mess. The tears were filling up my eyes when he said, "Do you think I give a FUCK about a fucking period?"

And to his point, men are nasty, and of course, yeah, they'll take any pussy they can get.

I shrugged, and he said, "Open your legs and hurry up." I sat flabbergasted because . . . I mean, did he really want me to leak all over his custom leather interior?

"NOW!" he ordered. I pulled my underwear to the side, trying to get the pad in my grip so he didn't look at it. He put two fingers inside me and brought them to his lips. He started to suck the blood off his index and middle fingers and licked his lips as if I had just made his favorite meal.

"Again," he said. I opened back up so he could get more blood on his hands, and he cleaned his wrist off as he proceeded through traffic. "I fucking love you. Do you know that? Do you see it now?"

Now, either your stomach is turning, or your heart is beating fast, but if that isn't excitement and mystery, I don't know what is!

The real test came when he met my mom. I moved my mom across the street from my LA apartment, so naturally, we headed over for dinner one night while he was visiting me. I was so nervous. I love her, but my mother is a hot fucking mess. Sometimes, she just has diarrhea of the mouth, and she knows it. She likes to blame it on being old, but, girl . . . YOU HAVE ALWAYS BEEN LIKE THIS.

She opened the door, and he gave her the biggest hug. They had small talk about the weather while I went to the bathroom.

Of course, I ear-hustled a little bit—because duh. I heard her say to him, "Thank you for making my daughter so happy."

His reply was fast, and he said, "She deserves it because she's an amazing woman." All I could see next was a white picket fence and a baby in our future.

But in April of 2024, I passed a pregnancy at home in my shower. I was shaking, throwing up, sick to my stomach about how this pain could be real. He held the shower curtain open to watch me and make sure I didn't pass out. When I stood upright, I felt something pouring out of me but couldn't look, and he saw it. He saw that stringy, dark, bloody sac that was somehow our month-old fetus. When I got out of the shower, I lay on the floor between his legs, and I cried so badly. He iced my arms, my neck, and my face. He held me and told me how sorry he was. How strong I was. How amazing I will be as a mother when we're ready.

I worried that this traumatic experience would be where the love stopped. I worried that finding out the size of my fibroid would affect our future fertility and our sex life. I called him, weeping about my ultrasound results where the nurse said I would probably never be able to have a vaginal birth. He listened to me, and for the first time, I heard the "WE."

"Baby, WE are going to figure this out. WE are going to have a healthy pregnancy one day. WE are going to have a successful birth. Because WE get everything WE want."

And I actually do believe that we can make anything happen. Because our love is so powerful that the hard times are not the end but a new kind of beginning.

I've finally progressed to the phase of life that I had been asking every psychic, Magic 8 Ball, and God for. I kept asking about the person I wanted: what they would look like, how tall they'd be, and how much money they would make. Actual growth taught me that this was a juvenile way of thinking. I should have always been asking for the mutual love that I deserved.

I not only asked for and manifested it, but I was ready to receive it. Now, I have it. Now, we have it.

Patriarchal Bullshit

"The whole education of women ought always to
have respect to the duties which they are to fulfil
towards men. They should be taught from their infancy
to please men; to be useful, and to make themselves beloved
and honoured by them; to bring them up from their youth;
to take care of them, when grown up; to advise, to console
them, and to render their life agreeable and pleasant;
these are the duties of women at all times."
—Jean-Jacques Rousseau (French philosopher and writer)[1]

Matriarchal Reply

"A man is absolutely not a necessity. . . .
I love men. I think men are the coolest.
But you don't really need them to live."
—Cher (singer and actress)[2]

WHY DO YOU NEED ME TO NEED YOU?

« MANDII B »

NOW, I KNOW that humans need certain things to live. We require the following basic necessities: water, food, air, and shelter. So it absolutely befuddles the hell out of me that the narrative for a cis woman is that in addition to those basic needs is the absolute NEED for a man. Don't get me wrong, I love a strong, confident, attractive, and well-endowed man like the rest of you who do. But do I NEED him? Where does the power lie in being dependent on or in NEED of another human being? A child needs their parents. A pet needs its caretaker. But do women really NEED men?

In classic Disney movies from our youth, the leading lady almost always falls head over heels for a man. And he was much more likely to love her in return if she needed to be rescued from her poor, unfortunate circumstances. Cinderella is saved from her awful living situation with her stepmom and stepsisters after the prince falls for her, the unattainable woman who runs away at the ball. He seeks out the woman who fits the glass slipper, and she is saved and becomes a princess. Ariel betrays her family, puts them all in danger, and gives up her voice to woo Eric. Belle falls in love with a controlling Beast and finds herself walking on eggshells and swallowing her pride as she deals with his mood swings and his clear mental trauma. Let's not forget Snow White, who a man saves not only from death, but from a poor situation of constantly cleaning after her seven male roommates because only women know how to clean up after a household. We have been programmed from early on that a man will most likely be our savior, our saving grace, protecting us from evil and freeing us from terrible living situations.

Ironically enough, this was the actual reality for us as women for a very long time. As far back as the Roman Empire, women were under the legal control of men, whether their fathers, husbands, or legal guardians (the *tutela mulierum perpetua*), who had to provide formal approval for certain legal acts, typically those involving property transfers. This system was somewhat reformed under Augustus, who enacted laws to encourage larger families. A woman who had given birth to at least three named children was allowed to become *sui iuris* (legally emancipated) upon divorce or the death of her husband. Wow, lucky her.

In Ancient Egypt, women theoretically shared the same legal rights and status as men. An Egyptian woman was entitled to own private property, which could include land, livestock, slaves, and servants. She had the right to inherit from others and to bequeath her belongings. Women could also divorce their husbands, reclaiming all their possessions, including the dowry. Additionally, they had the right to sue in court. If a husband beat his wife, he could be flogged and/or fined.[3] But the way that women were treated as equals in Egypt was certainly not the norm.

In the United States, it wasn't until the women's rights movement of the 1800s that women began making much more significant strides. In 1848, the Married Woman's Property Act was passed in New York. The act was subsequently used as a model for other states, all passing their versions by 1900.[4] With this act in place, a woman was no longer liable for her husband's debts, could enter into contracts on her own, collect rent or receive an inheritance in her own right, and file a lawsuit on her own behalf. But let's be very clear—this was just a baby step. Many women could not have their own bank accounts until 1974, when the Equal Credit Opportunity Act passed, which was supposed to prohibit credit discrimination. Before the passing of this act, many banks granted credit cards to women only with their husbands' signatures and outright refused to issue them to unmarried women.[5] For centuries, women couldn't make an affordable wage, vote, or be hired in a C-suite-level position.

So, based on history, did women NEED men? Abso-fucking-lutely. But with political and societal shifts, is this the case today? I say abso-fucking-lutely not. My last relationship with The Ex ended with this very argument.

Toward the tail end of a three-year less than perfect relationship driven by a person with many narcissistic tendencies, I found myself constantly trying to fix what he told me was wrong. We introduced ethical non-monogamy fairly early in our relationship. I craved women and wanted to share him with them. I introduced him to the lifestyle by bringing women into the bedroom for threesomes, making the nude beach a weekly summer activity, and attending sex clubs every month. Considering we were both new to ethical non-monogamy, we found ourselves customizing this uncharted world. We would close the relationship when we needed to focus more on ourselves. We'd communicate our feelings and only allow other parties to join us when we felt more comfortable. The problem was his inability to be honest, and that's a pretty big requirement when you're supposed to be ETHICAL in a non-monogamous relationship. He betrayed my trust repeatedly and found it easier to hide and lie about his other affairs, telling me I could not "handle the truth." He made decisions for the relationship I wouldn't have consented to.

I wonder how many of you can relate to this—being in a relationship where you are so in love that you begin to lose sight of who you are. And of who *they* really are.

Here are a few signs that you may be losing yourself in a relationship:

- You no longer prioritize your career.
- You are no longer into your hobbies or other special interests.
- You have lost touch with your friends and/or family because you are putting your romantic relationship first.
- You have lost your unique sparkle and shine.
- YOU are losing sight of YOU.

I'm not trying to make an excuse for my stupidity, but the toxicity of my relationship with The Ex took a while to spot. I met him during the pandemic via Zoom when the world literally shut down. He had no idea how successful I was because there was no way to measure my success when we were in our little bubble. Because of this, when things opened up, we had to navigate our time differently. Many things triggered his insecurities around my prosperity; the fact that I was a public figure and had a hectic travel schedule added to his paranoia.

An internal battle began; I wanted to love him unconditionally and be who he needed me to be. I also wanted to do what was necessary to continue climbing my ladder to success. As soon as work picked up for me, he scolded me for not cooking homemade meals anymore. Whenever I would travel, he would find ways to argue with me—hopping on a flight equated to hopping on some dick to him. His guilty conscience (yes, HE was cheating) made him believe I was cheating on him whenever I was out of town. When I reached career milestones, he would start arguments or give me the silent treatment. He threatened to break up so often that I saw the pattern. His absence from or need to start trouble in our relationship impacted how I celebrated my victories.

I remember walking through Washington Square Park, sipping bone broth as the trees began to get their color back and the flowers bloomed. He wore a bubble vest over his checkered button-up shirt, and I wore a light sweater and cargo jeans. Because of our differences in age, religious background, and understanding of how the world works, we constantly found ourselves in healthy debates about life. We would debate women's roles in the workplace vs. men, whether the Earth could really be flat, and whether or not Kanye West was really a genius or out of his mind.

I'm not even sure what prompted the following conversation, but once we opened this can, we never found a way to get everything back in it.

The Ex: You know women need men, right?

Me: SHIT! Women don't NEED men. They can be a great addition, but NEED? A woman can live and thrive without a man.

The Ex: So you don't need me?

Me: Ha! Hell nah, I don't need you. I want you. I choose you. But I don't NEED you.

Then there was silence. I don't think he believed my sentiment was genuine. This was the first time he heard it. He had already questioned his role and place in my life, but I thought my actions affirmed him, and my love was loud. I know my words stung him because this became an almost weekly debate until the end. There was a question about how we could exist in partnership without my need for him. I grew frustrated by this narrative.

Now check it: if you're a millennial, we can sit here and blame Ne-Yo for telling us an independent woman was the kind of girl he needed in his hit record "Miss Independent." Or perhaps we blame Destiny's Child for having us throw our hands in the air with pride for paying our own bills in their single "Independent Women Part I" on the *Charlie's Angels* soundtrack. Or maybe we blame rappers Webbie and Lil Boosie, who made sure we knew how to spell the word while we shouted out "I-N-D-E-P-E-N-D-E-N-T" with their 2008 smash. For many women, going to college, obtaining a degree, and being a boss became the goal. We changed our dreams of fairy-tale weddings and houses with white picket fences to dreams of traveling the world and becoming self-made.

I don't want to lose you here, so you should pause and ask yourself these three questions:

1. What three things bring the most joy to you, past or present?
2. When you were younger, what was the one idea that excited you the most about becoming an adult?
3. If you are currently in a relationship, what is the thing you fear the most that your partner could do to hurt you? If you are currently single, what is keeping you from being in a relationship?

Do not continue reading until you have locked in the answers to these questions.

I find it only fair to answer these questions myself so you can further understand my sentiments in this chapter:

1. My friends, traveling to new places, and accomplishing my goals (like writing this book)
2. Being able to do what I want when I want and to do it without needing anyone's permission
3. I'm alone, but I'm not lonely. I only want to welcome additions into my life that bring genuine happiness and joy. I'm open to finding love again, but not at the price of my peace.

I have been in weekly therapy for the past four years, and I recently realized that I experienced the mirror being held right in front of me, forcing me to dive into the depths of my own decision-making. Do you know what I NEEDED in the most profound moments of my insecurities? A man's validation to make me feel desired. Do you know what I NEEDED when I was struggling to pay my bills? A man's wallet to help me get over the hump. Do you know what I NEEDED in times of depression? A man's dick to numb me from reality and help me reach my orgasmic bliss, even if just temporarily. I found my NEED for men in my late teens and into my twenties to be pathetic and, honestly, quite embarrassing. Where was my dignity? Where was the value I held for myself? Could I not find happiness by being alone? Why did I seek out men to help me in all the areas I fell short in? I realized that I had put so much of myself into the hands of men that I inevitably lost Mandii.

Back to that conversation in Washington Square Park: I broke the silence and finally told The Ex about my trauma. I told him that I had negative associations with the word "NEED." I had needed men in my past for things that, in hindsight, brought me shame. I was so proud of myself to finally be in a relationship with a man that I CHOSE. I told him, "I choose to be with you because I want and love you." For the first time, I felt empowered being with someone I genuinely enjoyed being around, cared for, and deeply loved without the transactional focus on tangible items. This was nothing like any other relationship I'd had with a man. My previous interactions with them now seemed desperate. The transactional nature of needing them to be a Band-Aid over whatever scar I couldn't heal alone was pathetic. My reliance on their funds to eat, pay bills, and travel the world was despicable. There was a codependency between them wanting to have sex with me for their pleasure and me somehow conflating that desire with a false sense of validation about my worth and beauty. I even see my relationship with my father as somewhat transactional because he guilted me into feeling as though I were indebted to him for the child support payments he made.

When I got into this relationship, my very first relationship as an adult, I only felt comfortable doing so because I was finally ready to show up for a partner in a way I hadn't felt adequate enough to do before. The pounds that kept me insecure in my own skin had been shed. The money I was once lacking, I now had in abundance. I'd also gotten to a place of sexual freedom where I could be myself and share all of my desires with my partner without shame.

I had to deprogram my thoughts from being a side chick for a third of my life. I had learned to jump through the mental hoops of my trauma that constantly kept me from getting what I wanted out of a man. I had to lean into knowing that I could make plans, demand that someone see me more often, and hold them accountable for how their actions made me feel. My feelings finally mattered, and how I wanted a man to show up for me could be effectively communicated. I no longer had to take the crumbs that a man was throwing at me and could now have the whole damn cake. I didn't care about how much money he gave me because this relationship was built on a foundation that went beyond a financial transaction. I was no longer in survival mode or looking for a knight in shining armor to save me. Choosing a partner looked like how I chose my closest friends. I felt safe to share my secrets. I looked forward to making plans, exploring new places, and creating memories together. This feeling made me never want to return to the pits of hell and NEED a man to feel whole.

I shared the premise of this chapter with my close friend, and she threw a hypothetical question at me that hit me like a bag of bricks: "What if he'd told you that he didn't NEED you? How would that have made you feel?"

My heart sank immediately. I'm unsure why, but I gasped and felt hurt. It didn't feel too good to hear, maybe because I was putting myself in the same shoes I'd put my partner in. My immediate reaction was the feeling of unworthiness and sadness. I repeated the question to myself and snapped out of it. I thought of every way I was capable and how I chose to show up in a relationship with a partner. I also connected it to my decision to not have kids. I even thought about my being a cat owner over a dog owner. The connection to the word "NEED" and the idea of a man NEEDING me switched my emotional gears off, and I answered the question logically. I would love a partner who also CHOOSES me and doesn't necessarily NEED me. I want to know that we come together to make each other better, not to try and make one another whole. However, on our own, we can also thrive and be great versions of ourselves. Without me, he can live independently, feed himself, and be a great human being; however, he'd rather do these things WITH ME. CHOOSING to be with someone is what looks like love to me.

I realized that my views on needing a man made me feel like I was sacrificing or giving away my control. Battling this notion, I called on a close professional colleague to help me flesh out my thoughts. Am I in such dire need of control that my views on needing a man bother me? He shared the following analogy with me and created an AHA! moment of clarity.

If you want to make a potato salad, you'll need certain ingredients. A simple recipe will need potatoes, hard-boiled eggs, seasonings, pickled relish, veggies, and mayonnaise. Your choice becomes which kind of mayonnaise you want. Are you choosing Miracle Whip, Hellmann's, Duke's, or the value brand? Regardless of which brand you choose, mayo is necessary to create the potato salad that you want.

A relationship consists of two individuals who choose to be in a relationship. Therefore, if you want and desire to be in a relationship, another person is needed to complete the recipe.

Instead of reacting to my moment of complete honesty and baring my soul, The Ex chose to make it the literal end of everything. He simply could not accept that I did not NEED him but that I WANTED him. I would not back down from my stance. He knew what I'd experienced in my past. There were so many other red flags waving that our relationship had to end, but ultimately, this was one of the reasons he cited as the breaking point for him. Ironically, I began finding out that he'd cheated on me with a homeless girl and a mentally emotional wreck of another woman, both of whom he confirmed he felt affirmed by because they NEEDED him. If he could not understand the gift that I gave him by choosing him above all others, he probably did not deserve me. So we went our separate ways, and our breakup is the gift that keeps on giving. This breakup pushed me to learn about myself and grow through the pain.

DOES CLOSURE EVEN EXIST?

After ending that relationship, I spiraled into a deep depression. There was no more back-and-forth—it was truly over. He broke my heart and left me feeling betrayed with countless unanswered questions. For an entire year after the breakup, I dealt with an overwhelming sense of PTSD. Now, I know we usually associate that term with people who've been through war, but let me tell you, I didn't realize how much emotional damage I had endured. My body would almost shut down if a man were anywhere near me, and I even burst into tears when a guy simply asked if I wanted a massage.

I found myself apologizing for being on my phone around new partners, and certain conversations would instantly trigger me. Flashbacks of the gaslighting I endured would flood in, and I began feeling unsafe around men in general. Psychologically, I was shattered, and it took a tremendous amount of work to piece myself back together enough to consider being open to the idea of a new relationship. I decided to decenter sex for a while and spent time talking things through with my therapist, booking more sessions than I'd ever anticipated. I battled with the idea that none of the love I had experienced in that relationship was real, and I struggled with accepting the possibility of genuine love in the future. I needed closure, but I had no idea what that would even look like.

It was a Thursday afternoon in Harlem, and I had just left the funeral service of my friend and former manager, Jason. The two weeks leading up to the service had me on an emotional roller coaster. His death was sudden and unexpected, and I constantly found myself wiping away tears, thinking about all the memories we shared. This was the first time I experienced the death of someone I had recently made plans with—someone I had just been with, singing at the top of our lungs and messing up the lyrics.

After the service, I headed across the street with some friends who were also grieving, and we shared a quiet moment over lunch. We bonded through our mutual feelings of loss, filling our stomachs with comforting soul food at the famous Amy Ruth's on 116th Street. We were emotionally spent, so we decided to grab a drink to decompress and take a breather. But as soon as I stepped out of the bar, my heart dropped, just like that day in the park. There it was—my ex's truck, double-parked outside. I knew it was his; he was never one to follow traffic laws.

The liquid courage mixed with my swirling emotions pushed me to confront him. As soon as the headlights flicked on, I stormed toward the passenger side of his truck, my fist aggressively pounding on the window. When he turned toward me, startled, I instinctively threw up my middle finger and then backed away toward the rear of his car, my heart racing. What happened next wasn't at all how I'd imagined our first encounter would go if we ever crossed paths again. He stepped out of the driver's seat, angry and equally confused. "Why did you bang on my window?" he demanded, his voice matching his expression. We locked eyes, and in that moment, my anger melted away, replaced by a wave of overwhelming sadness. I felt hollow, like the weight of grief, sorrow, and despair had crashed over me all at once. I was still raw from losing my friend, and now every unresolved emotion related to our breakup hit me. With my voice shaking, I finally let out what had been trapped inside me for so long. "You fucked me up. You hurt me so bad. But you REALLY fucked me up."

That's all I could keep repeating to him: "You really fucked me up." I didn't cry—not because I didn't want to, but because I had already cried every tear I had over the last two weeks, and especially that morning. Deep down, I wanted to scream all the questions I'd been holding in since the end of our relationship. Why did he cheat on me with those other women? Why wasn't I enough? Why couldn't he be honest with me? Did I not create a safe space for him? Was I a bad partner? Was anything we had even real?

To my surprise, we agreed to meet up later that night at a lounge in Soho to talk in depth. We parted ways after standing there in the street, and just before saying goodbye, I leaned in for a hug. I needed that hug—needed the comfort and the feeling of being held. That desire for warmth, for something familiar, is what led me to cancel on him just ten minutes before we were supposed to meet. I couldn't go through with it. After talking to my friends and even my mother, they all said the same thing: *Don't do it!* I was ready to ignore their advice, meet him, and take this secret to the grave. But something in me shifted. My gut told me to stop.

If I'm being honest, I didn't just want a hug—I wanted him deep inside me. I was craving affection, intimacy, and, yeah, some dick. I was a vulnerable, emotional wreck. But as I stood on the platform waiting for the train to take me to him, I turned around. I knew I wasn't in any state to risk adding REJECTION to the mess of emotions I was already dealing with. What if he didn't want me like that anymore? What if he didn't give me the safety and warmth I so desperately needed? And what if I woke up the next morning wondering why I had opened up old wounds for nothing? I didn't need the weight of REGRET on top of mourning.

I called him while he was circling the area, searching for parking. I repeated what I had said in the text I'd sent moments earlier, explaining that I wasn't strong enough to be in his presence that night.

Instead of meeting up, we ended up having a two-and-a-half-hour conversation over the phone. Every emotion, thought, concern, and memory we had been holding on to poured out. We talked through the highs and lows of our roller-coaster relationship, unpacking all the sharp turns and dips. It was eye-opening to realize how differently we had weighed certain moments, but by the end, we both came to the same conclusion—what we had was real.

The next morning, I woke up feeling lighter, like a weight had been lifted off my chest. *Was this what closure felt like?* Rolling over, I grabbed my phone and texted him to express my gratitude for our conversation the night before.

Moments later, his response came through. When he saw me, he thought he'd be ready with all the right words, but when the moment came, he froze—all the things he'd planned to say disappeared.

He said that realizing I didn't hate him surprised him the most. He admitted he deserved to be hated after everything that happened. But when he got out of his truck, he saw something he wasn't prepared for in my face—a softness and a warmth that caught him off guard. He said he knew I had one of the kindest hearts of anyone he'd been with, even if it was wrapped in a protective layer.

He thanked me for letting him speak his mind, say what he felt, and apologize for how he'd hurt me. He finally admitted he'd used his words as weapons, trying to match my wit to avoid taking accountability for his actions.

He even talked about all the times he'd traveled across the city trying to keep our connection alive. He told me it was all too wild, beautiful, sometimes painful, and impossible to forget. I appreciated him saying I am "truly one of a kind."

And then he topped it off by saying he was sorry for letting me down.

Closure in a relationship can look different for everyone, but all in all, it's acceptance of the end and the peace to move forward. While I may not know precisely what I want from a partner, I do know that I desire to be in a relationship. Within navigating my bisexuality, I understand that I enjoy sexual relationships with women without the desire to be in a romantic, committed relationship with one. I've always known that my romantic relationship would exist with a man. I don't picture myself having children or walking down an aisle to be wed. However, I do WANT to be in a long-term and committed relationship.

When I am in my next relationship, it will be with someone who comprehends that if I CHOOSE them as my partner, that is my way of showing them that I love them. If I find someone who has "all the things" on their own and they CHOOSE to be with me, what an honor that would be. Life keeps coming, so I am not saying there may not be a time when one of us needs more support than the other. I would only ask that if I lend them a hand when they are down, they will do the same for me. No questions asked, because we will CHOOSE one another through the good and the bad. And as long as this relationship continues to be something we keep on CHOOSING, I will stay. But if it ever shifts to a space of desperation where I NEED them or they NEED me, I will have to CHOOSE ME.

To me, love is a choice. Right now, I CHOOSE to love myself. I get up every morning and thank God for the life I have created with his blessing. And I will wait until I find the man who will love me the way I love him. I hope that he is out there because, to be honest, this girl's damn patience is running out. But for today, I CHOOSE Mandii, because she is the only person I actually NEED.

Patriarchal Bullshit

"I don't understand how me asking for casual sex is such a
wild concept for you to grasp. Aren't you from New York?"
—Random Asshole from Bumble that
Weezy went out on two dates with circa 2017

Matriarchal Reply

"So maybe it won't look like you thought it would
in high school, but it's important to remember that
love is possible. Anything is possible. This is New York."
—Carrie (Sarah Jessica Parker's character in
Sex and the City)[1]

IF 9 MILLION PEOPLE ARE HERE, WHY DO I FEEL ALONE?*

« WEEZYWTF »

NOT SAYING I'M one of those weirdos from TV that wants to fuck a car or something (I'm not trying to kink-shame), but I did fall in love with something that isn't a person. I fell for a place. I fell madly, deeply, and passionately in love with New York because of everything she has given to me. Like a person, loving a city—especially when it's not working—takes real commitment and care. Like any relationship, you must put in the time, nurture it, and stick around through the highs and lows. It can push you, make you grow, and challenge you in ways you didn't expect—just like the best relationships do. Now, everyone already knows New York is the shit, but the stuff that actually sucks? It's not the rats, the smell of pee, or even the sky-high rent.

While the city brought out the best in me, it's also unleashed some of my worst. Throughout my time here, I've fluctuated between moments of growth and bouts of depression, all because of her EXTREMES. Everything here is dialed up—the constant need for cash, the weather you can't escape, the never-ending stress—but the loneliness really hit me hardest.

I've told you I'm originally a Florida girl—not the rednecky alligator-eatin' kind, just a transplant whose parents wanted a better life in a cheaper place. I never felt at home in Orlando. I know that Mandii talked in her chapters about some of the biases many Floridians seem to have. I have to concur; I always had people gossiping behind my back about my bisexuality, saying that I was a slut, or whatever name they felt like using for a woman who carried the confidence they lacked! I was always able to be free even in a town with limitations, but not being around your tribespeople can be exhausting. I always knew I'd be leaving, but I finally took the plunge at twenty-five years old.

New York became where I could be myself, no apologies. Here, you can casually mention you're bi, and people barely blink, like, "And...?" If anything, this city offers experiences you can't get anywhere else. But she's also dangerous. Thinking back, I'm lucky I'm still here to tell some of these tales.

It's wild to feel so empty in one of the most populated cities in the world. And when you feel lonely and disconnected, it leads you to make questionable choices to connect. Okay, sometimes I just wanted a good fuck, but sometimes I made these less than stellar decisions because I was trying to fill the void or numb the fuck out.

How much do you matter when you're one of 9 million people? You're surrounded by humans but still feel entirely unseen. As a total transplant with no friends or community when I first arrived, I was just trying to figure it the fuck out. Loneliness became the biggest test of who I am. It was like the city held up a mirror and demanded, "Now that you're here, WHO ARE YOU?" The constant feeling of being insignificant can really kick your ass.

They say you can never have all three things at once: a good job, a good apartment, and a good love. In my case, I never thought I'd get a partner, let alone LOVE somebody in New York. As non-monogamous as I can be, the catch-22 is that when you're in a place filled with so many options, sometimes "an option" is all you become, too.

This is a place where models walk around like regular civilians, passing by the man of your dreams as a reminder that he doesn't want to settle down or text your short self back. A place where you can grab a latte at your local coffee shop, run into an investment banker who happens to need a plus-one for his Hampton weekend trip, and boom . . . Your bitch is gone!

Seeing how easy it was for people to have experiences like these gave me less faith and hope in meeting someone to "love." It became difficult for me to stop comparing myself because I sank more into loneliness every time I walked out the door. But I had the perfect cure for my pity party:

THE DATING APPS.

The place where loneliness goes away. The place where, with the click of your messages, you're reminded how hot you are by every douchebag that wants to get into your pants for the night. We all *know* that is the only thing they're usually looking for, but the 1 percent chance that I'd meet the ONE who's actually looking for love and commitment is what kept me swiping.

Location: Weezy's desk, 1 Park Ave
Time: Noonish

Me: Left, left, left, left, so far left, left, left, left.

Hmm, maybe, right? Ew, look at those dirty fin-
gernails. LEFT.

Left, left, left, left, left.

Ugh, a big fish pic?!? Seriously? Left.

Left, left, ooh!

He's cute! Shit, is that his baby? Left.

Those were the thoughts of my daily swiping—my favorite "on-
the-clock" pastime! I never ran out of men because my girl, New
York, has millions of them to go through—plus the international
hotties looking for a city girl to show them a good time. And there I
was, the perfect welcome wagon!

He was 6'6", Australian, and beefy! Not my usual type, but he
was so fine I just had to swipe right. An instant match? Of course.

We met up at Totto Ramen. I was there first, and I remember
him having to duck his head down to enter the spot.

HE. WAS. HUGE.

I can't remember what exact job he was in town for, but it
should've been football.

We had a nice exchange and shared some banter over sake before
he finally said, "All right, let's figure out how you're going to get out
of this, young lady." He pointed to my phone and said, "Come on,
then, let's prepare your excuse for missing work tomorrow."

What I thought: *Is he literally fucking insane? Typical douchebag.
Men expect you to cave and do whatever the fuck it is that THEY desire
at the expense of your LIVELIHOOD. A man I have known for one hour
expects me to take the chance and risk my JOB just so I can spend the night
with him.*

What I did: I immediately unlocked my phone, opened the mail app, and drafted an email to my boss with him over the remaining sake. Once it was sent through, he said, "YEAH! THERE WE GO! LET'S FUCK SHIT UP!" Did I tell you that I am a pushover when it comes to men this hot and tall with an accent?

We jumped on Citi Bikes and soared off into the night.

Weezy and whatever-his-name-is's timeline went something like this:

11:20 p.m.—Make out session in Central Park

11:40 p.m.—Still in Central Park, buy molly from a random guy

12:00 a.m.—A subway ride to Bushwick

12:40 a.m.—House of Yes? YES!

1:10 a.m.— . . . okay, this is too much, next!

1:30 a.m.—Weird underground jazz bar. Where are we?

3:00 a.m.—Pizza!!!

3:45 a.m.—The pizza is good, but should we take a little of the molly we got from that weird guy in Central Park?

4:45 a.m.—Okay, it's fully kicked in; what the fuck??? Why would we do this???

6:00 a.m.—My feet hurt. We head back to his place.

He put the key in the lock right around the time the sun appeared. The two of us swallowed each other's faces. In my mind, we were straight out of a movie. I don't know how we got there, but not many words were exchanged. Sometimes the nonverbal cues are even sexier than the actual sex itself, and I find that I would prefer knowing you wanna fuck me by just looking you in the eye than hearing you tell me.

He went into the kitchen to pour a shot. I followed behind him and jumped up onto the countertop. I pulled my tank top over my head and pushed my titties together, so he had a special shot holder. He laughed, put the glass in between my breasts, and used his mouth to shoot it back.

There was tequila all over me, and he cleaned up every single drop. As he licked me around my waist, sucking up all the remaining liquor mixed with my sweat, he kept making this weird but supremely hot moaning noise. The kind of noise you make when you're eating something really tasty. Not tryna toot my horn, but . . . Yes, I am. BEEP BEEP.

Still with no words exchanged, we rolled around the living room floor, laughing about how silly we felt with each tumble or bump into each other's teeth. He started to lick me, almost like a lollipop, in this weird (but oddly sexy) disgusting way. Like he was cleaning me up. He finally made his way onto my pussy lips. I felt a rush of insecurity because I hadn't done my usual hoe bath after a night out, but fuck it, let him enjoy the sweat! It felt so barbaric in a way; he used his teeth and made me watch him as he kept saying, "LOOK AT ME!" I was so horny from all of the night's foreplay I begged him to get a condom.

With his head between my legs, he said, "Shit, I don't have one."

Now, in this scenario, most men will try to fuck you anyway, but I appreciate that he didn't. He stood up with a rock-hard dick, lookin' around random places, and shouted about how he should've just gotten a damn hotel.

I had the grand idea of ordering condoms from Uber Eats, popped open the app, got a pack of rubbers and some chips, and updated him on the twenty-minute ETA.

"Fuck, I love New York!" he said.

"Well . . . what shall we do to pass the time?"

He tried to get back between my legs, but to be honest, I was gettin' way too turned on; I felt like I may just take a chance on the nameless foreigner and make him put that thick raw dick inside of me. I told him, "I can't handle it . . . but I would love to tease you."

I suggested mutual masturbation.

It may sound juvenile, but it was one of the sexiest scenarios I've been in. We both got naked and sat facing each other on the couch. I let him use a little of my saliva as lube for himself before I lay back on my end so he could get the perfect view of my pretty pussy. He locked eyes with me, stroking his dick while telling me exactly what he wanted to see.

"Put one finger inside. Wait, now put it in your mouth and lick off the cream . . . stick out your tongue and show me."

Damn, he was nasty!!! And we still had eleven minutes to go!

This. Shit. Was. Sexy!!!

We kept pleasing ourselves, using our free hands for encouragement and doing our best to give a grand show. I was watching the precum ooze out of his dick while he kept promising to hold his cum for me. I was so committed to making him break his edge that I shot my spit onto his dick from my position on the couch, and he moaned just feeling it land on him. The delivery driver arrived during our nastiness, and we both screamed, "YOU CAN LEAVE IT!" as he knocked.

Laughing at our persistence, we took a break and lay naked next to each other. I wish I could give you the sex details, but it wasn't really as memorable as the masturbation. We fell asleep, woke up to fool around some more, and I wore his clothes downstairs as he called his cab. Apparently, he wanted me to keep a piece of him, but I just wanted the free hoodie.

When he was leaving, he looked at me and said that he wanted to tell me he loved me. He felt an intensity for me like he had never felt with someone else. He quickly followed that up with "Or maybe it's just New York."

I wasn't offended because the feeling was mutual.

My twenty-four-hour love affair was a real thing born from the isolation and sadness the city brought me. This place where people are so often dicks that you suspect any compliment to be a setup. It's so hard not to fucking cling to anyone or anything that finally pays attention to you, even if it is a little bit of fake love.

Getting my fix of that love was becoming an obsession. It wasn't just us women who felt alone. It was the men, too! And boy, does the feeling of loneliness meet its PEAK in wintertime. Just like the bears hibernate, so do the people. Cuffin' season arrives, and those of us who didn't get chosen are home stuffing our faces and watching reruns.

This led to another day of swiping for me since I had nothing better to do on days when the snow was so high that you could barely see in front of you. A blizzard was happening—the first I had ever experienced. TV told everyone to stock up, kids couldn't go to school, and grocery stores were closing for the storm. As insane as it sounds, I still wanted to get into trouble, and I knew that swiping would get me there.

This time, it was a DJ. He was kinda awkward-looking, but according to my friends, I've been known to fuck an ugly guy or two.

Immediately upon matching, he sent me a message: "Come to Williamsburg tonight. I'm DJ'ing." My initial thought was always to try to get dinner, drinks, or a little effort first, but there was a massive snow apocalypse . . . and like I said, the loneliness was setting in. I didn't know what to expect, but at least it was at Baby's All Right, a spot in Williamsburg I was familiar with.

When I arrived, he was at the turntables and sweating like he'd just finished a 5K. We said hello, he offered me some molly, and I quickly declined. *What the fuck?* I thought to myself, he doesn't even know how to pronounce my name yet. After about an hour of watching him do it and making sure the drug wouldn't kill me, I figured, fuck it, why not? (Safety win?!? Eh?!?)

I told him to mix the molly with some water for me, and he obliged. While DJing, he made a little mixture and set up four empty shot glasses for us and his friends. Since the taste of molly is fucking disgusting, I shot the whole glass to get it over with.

In the middle of the transition to a different song, he shouted, "YO. THAT WAS SUPPOSED TO BE FOR ALL OF US."

Turns out the four shot glasses were to be split up among everyone, and now I'd had four times the average dose of MDMA on an 18-degree night during a snowstorm, with a guy I'd just met. GREAT!

I rushed downstairs and threw it up with the help of one of his friends who came down and offered to be my "drug coach." I got over it and felt better after an hour. I shared a fun dance with Tinder guy, and honestly, the euphoric sensation that you're supposed to feel . . . set in! He asked if I wanted to come back to his loft to keep hanging out, and I said yes.

When we got into the cab, the drug started to wear off, and I remember feeling a bit sad as I came down. The snow was tinged with black soot, and I got to SEE New York in her ugly. She seemed to match the path I was taking for myself. I didn't even necessarily find the DJ attractive, but the warmth of his thigh touching mine, the attention, and the affection made me feel more whole than I'd felt alone in my place. We walked into his apartment, and there was a woman there crying. She happened to be one of his roommates (yes, in a LOFT) and was in tears about a man who she said was making her consider relapsing. When I asked on what, she replied, "HEROIN."

Now I know I do some shit, but shooting up is MY hard no and time to kink-shame. *Bitch, how the FUCK did you end up with these crazy-ass white people?* I thought to myself. I continued to sip on whatever drink they made me and just enjoy these crazy stories since I planned on never seeing him again anyway.

As the MDMA faded more, the serotonin was leaving my body, and I desperately wanted to stop feeling the comedown. I asked if he had any Benadryl or something I could take to sleep; he handed me a bag of mixed narcotics and told me to find a Xanax. After searching through the pill identifier website, he finally identified a relaxant that we both took.

As our bodies got heavier and it was time to go to sleep, I went up some tiny stairs into this little cocoon in the loft and crawled into his bed. I had drunk tons of water to try and sober up when we got in the house, and I started to feel the pressure on my bladder. We were lying down and cuddling when I asked him to help me down the stairs to pee.

"Ah man, I can't move, either, though . . . so just pee right here."

THIS NIGGA WAS REALLY FUCKING CRAZY.

We were lying IN HIS BED! And honestly, I wanna tell you that I didn't do it, but I don't fucking remember. I woke up somewhere around 4 p.m., and the trains were finally running. After opening my eyes to a weird-ass room, feeling and SMELLING awful, I left him without saying goodbye and took the forty-five-minute ride home, wondering if what I'd done was epic or just downright disgusting. I'm pretty sure it's the latter.

Talking about this wild night on episode 4 of *WHOREible De-*

cisions became one of the most popular stories, but later, I came to regret it. I realized how ridiculous I was for trying to stay out of actual solitude. As funny as the story is, I had to collect myself and ask *why* I put myself into these dumb-ass predicaments. It's because I was running. I continued to run away from that mirror New York was showing me instead of looking into it. I call it the "pee story" in jest, but in reality, it's the story of when I was so desperate for company that I put my literal life in jeopardy. I took some random prescription meds from a total fucking stranger, not even for the fun of it but just to escape that sadness. The reality is that I never knew how to lean in until I was forced to.

My first year in the city was incredible. I had a big luxury two-bedroom apartment in Midtown, a year's worth of rent paid by my sugar daddy, twenty-five pounds less on the scale, and a hangover bounce-back like you've never seen. I was living life like a *true* transplant with no repercussions or sense of how grimy this place really was. My beer goggles came off around twenty-six during my second year.

The second winter felt COLDER. It wasn't much fun when you weren't going on some random date with a DJ from Brooklyn . . . I could FEEL everything. I would wake up for work at 6 a.m. when it was dark outside and leave by 5 p.m. when it was *again* dark outside. I would return home to my new apartment on the Lower East Side, which was 312 square feet. I lived at 150 Orchard, on the top floor of a building that only offered studios. I was surrounded by action but had no energy or will to get up. I took my winter clothes off in the same place every day and went right to bed, which became my dining table, desk, and confessional. I ate all my meals on the top of my comforter, watching the same episodes of the same shows because the anxiety of what would happen on a new show felt like too much. I wouldn't say I liked how I talked to myself, how I thought about myself, and how I would pick apart all the flaws in my body. The discoloration on my neck, the eczema, the thickness of my hair, all of it. EEW. I hated being me.

Even though the apartment was small, getting up to use the bathroom felt like scaling Mount Everest. I would lie in bed wondering if dying in my sleep would feel more comfortable than forcing myself to get up. Dying . . . I would fantasize about ways it could happen quickly without pain. Sometimes it would be a tortuous game in my head of objects I would do it with. Knife. Pills. Hammer. Fumes. Whatever was in my line of sight from my bed, I would obsess about it.

The day I planned to do it, I called out of work. I went outside in the freezing cold of January to spend some much-needed time with New York before I left her. But I couldn't see anything in the depth of all that snow, so it didn't matter anyway. It was the type of cold that was so uncomfortable that your eyelashes were getting icy. I got myself a slice of pizza, watched *Sex and the City*, and found an old bottle of Valium that my mom had left accidentally after hip surgery. I googled how many pills I would need for it to work. Somehow, the algorithm was trying to talk me out of death. The frustrating thing was that all the marketing said "YOU ARE NOT ALONE." But yes, I was!!! Nobody was physically there. Sure, maybe a friend would have come over if I asked, but it was too embarrassing to talk about. I had always been the happy girl, and the shame from what I was feeling was so fucking heavy. I was about a year into the podcast, which felt like a place of comfort and liberation for women. How could I be the depressed girl who preaches for you to get out there and be happy?

I took three of the Valium to start. I was waiting for my heart to slow down until I took the rest. I had read somewhere that many people throw it all up, so I wanted to make sure that I did it right; throwing up all night would be way fuckin' worse than dying. After twenty minutes, my vision started to blur. I would describe it as almost like a mushroom high. Colors began to blend, and I laughed at every shape I started to see. It was the first time I had genuinely laughed in months. I started to hear New York noises; people yelling, music, loud horns, and it hit me that . . . I wasn't finished!

I called my friend Gilah, who lived a few blocks over, made up a lie about a bug in my apartment, and asked her if I could sleep over. She groaned and said, "Yes." I threw a coat on to hurry up and get there before I changed my mind. This may have been the most unorthodox way *not to die*, but in my mind, it made sense. I knew that if I was around someone I loved, I would never want them to have to watch me suffer. When this feeling of slight happiness went away, what if I took the rest of the pills? I knew sleeping on Gilah's couch that night would keep me here for another day. Her presence in the next room gave me a sense of responsibility over my life, which worked. In the morning, I told my therapist how bad my thoughts had gotten, and he prescribed me Lexapro.

I stayed on a drug that made me feel like a fucking robot, but at least I wasn't dead . . . I guess? The weird effect that antidepressants have on your body can affect your sex life. Even though I was a lonely gal with no partners, I'd always had a sex life by myself! I would masturbate for hours with my hands, toys, the end of a fuckin' hairbrush, vibrating toothbrush, anything! I still couldn't cum. Lexapro was hell.

After a few months, my therapist asked me how I was feeling, and I said, "Man, I mean, I don't really want to die anymore, but honestly, not being able to cum kinda makes me wanna kill myself."

He told me that he thought my joke was funny as hell but also had an inclination that I was "back."

Years go by, therapy happens, and a montage of reminders that the company of myself isn't a bad thing. I learned to get into situations that helped me plug into the noise instead of finding ways to avoid it. I am holding myself accountable to become the savvy New York City woman I always dreamed I would be.

You know her. She's the one who knows which museum has a fabulous new exhibit, tells you with conviction why biking is better than taking the train, or shares what places she discovered on a walk around her neighborhood. That, to me, is the New Yorker who understands how to operate without anyone. The only way to become her was to copy everything my ideal person would do. The way she would sound, walk, and dress.

After a while, all of my negative thoughts turned into mantras with a silver lining. Sentences like "I hate that I'm single" became "New York is the EASIEST place to be single!"

How could it not be when every night there was a free event, a gallery opening, a concert, a meetup group, or even a date with someone from the apps (when it's healthy and safe)?

Like every person who needs to "find themselves," I did my rounds of therapy. After shelling out tens of thousands of dollars to talk about how my childhood inflicted all of these wounds, my favorite therapy tactic I applied was how to change my automatic thoughts. My therapist had me set reminders and alarms on my phone with random messages that I *wanted* to believe so that it would eventually be normal to read.

I am worthy.

I am beautiful.

Most importantly, I am LOVED. Even when I am not in a romantic partnership.

Avoiding loneliness will only cause issues when you are finally sharing space. Growing mindfulness is vital to your overall self-esteem, productivity, and energy levels. Your brain starts to recover without all the external stimuli that this clusterfuck of a city brings. Yes, community and companionship are necessary, but so is being able to say you can be happy by yourself.

I finally realized that the most beautiful version of YOU doesn't arrive until you meet the ugliest you. So, thank you, NYC. Because I see how fuckin' hot I am now.

HELP IS AVAILABLE

The 988 Suicide & Crisis Lifeline understands that life's challenges can be hard. Whether you're facing mental health struggles, emotional distress, alcohol or drug use, or just need someone to talk to, their caring counselors are there for you. You are NEVER alone.

Call: 988

Visit: 988Lifeline.org

POWER

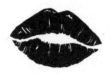

You can find your power only through making progress.

We can discover our power by embracing our strengths
and letting go of self-doubt. Finding your power
requires self-awareness, confidence, and courage.
When we recognize and own our abilities, we tap into
the core of who we are, unlocking the energy and potential
that have always been within us. Embracing our power
means standing firm in our beliefs and trusting ourselves,
allowing us to navigate life's challenges with purpose and clarity.
Through this process, we empower ourselves and
inspire and uplift those around us.

YOU finding YOUR POWER is the entire reason we created this book.

HOW DO WE DEFINE POWER?

« MANDII B + WEEZYWTF »

POWER THROUGH REFLECTION AND ACCOUNTABILITY

If you're reading this book, it's essential to acknowledge that each of us carries a past, lives in our present, and faces a future. As the saying goes, "History repeats itself." To truly gain power over your mind, spirit, and life, it is essential to look inward, confront your own faults, and hold yourself accountable. Yes, this means placing blame where it's due—on yourself—but more importantly, it also means forgiving yourself for those mistakes. Maybe you didn't have the tools or knowledge to make the correct decisions in the past, and that's okay. We don't always get things right on the first try. But understand this: there is no strength in ignorance or endless self-blame. The real power comes from acknowledging your missteps, correcting course, and growing from the experience.

ACCESSING POWER BY
REMOVING YOURSELF FROM VICTIMHOOD

There's immense strength in reclaiming your narrative and taking the power away from those who have caused you pain or trauma. Writing this book allowed us to take our power back by sharing our truths. Let's be honest—hurt people hurt people, and some genuinely awful individuals are in this world. We only get one life, so it is our job to permit ourselves to heal so that we can make the most of it. Power comes from shifting your mentality from victim to SURVIVOR. It's not about pretending the pain didn't happen but about refusing to let it define your future. Power is forgiving both yourself and your perpetrator, no matter how difficult that may seem. Now that you've read our stories, you know that we understand how damn hard that can be. The key is transforming your perspective: life isn't happening *to* you, it's happening *for* you. This shift can be life-altering, leading you from a place of suffering to one of empowerment. And as far as we can tell, that is the whole damn point of being here on Earth.

THE POWER OF RESILIENCE THROUGH APPRECIATION

Power is the ability to rise up, dust yourself off, and declare, "Never again." It's finding the courage to overcome adversity and open yourself up to life's beauty and magnificence, even in the smallest moments. This could mean connecting deeply with a friend, witnessing the simple beauty in nature, relaxing, or really feeling that mind-blowing orgasm deep down in your body. Take the time to appreciate the little things by stopping the noise outside yourself and listening. These moments of stillness allow you to reconnect. Put down your phone, stop scrolling, and get in touch with your inner self, God, Creator, or whatever higher force guides you. When you give yourself the space to appreciate these wonders, you give yourself a gift beyond measure—the gift of presence.

TRUSTING YOUR INNER POWER

Trusting yourself is a cornerstone of true power. This means listening to your intuition the first time it raises a red flag because your inner guide is rarely wrong. This level of self-trust requires a shift in attitude, understanding that your power lies in your ability to love and respect yourself fully. Throughout this book, we've shared moments of struggle—times when we lost self-respect or have allowed others to mistreat us. In those moments, we gave our power away. But in sharing these moments with you, we hope you'll see that true evolution comes from learning to love yourself and believing you deserve all the good things life has to offer—not just saying it but deeply believing this is true. Real power is knowing that other people's opinions shouldn't define how you feel about yourself. Self-love is where it's at.

OWNING YOUR UNIQUE SUPERPOWER

The truth is the power is within you. Only YOU get to define how powerful you are. Everyone has power, but some people have learned to harness and wield theirs more effectively. Those who seem the most "powerful" aren't necessarily the wealthiest or most successful individuals—they're often the ones who have the confidence to exist as their truest, most authentic selves, no matter who they're around. It's not about conforming but about maintaining authenticity across all spaces. Don't let anyone convince you to dim your light or make you doubt your own superpowers. The real strength isn't about how you're flexing on the outside, it's about the vibe and mindset you have on the inside.

Your true power is as unique as your fingerprint; no two are alike. It's about becoming the kind of person others are drawn to, who builds others up, is honest, and has figured out what brings them joy. Power is the quiet confidence of someone who knows exactly who they are and isn't afraid to embrace it. You are magnetic when you are in the flow and living your life authentically.

THE TRUE MEANING OF YOUR POWER

Ultimately, power isn't about money, status, or external success. It's about character, and being the kind of person who lifts others up rather than seeking to elevate themselves at the expense of others. True power comes from discovering what brings you genuine happiness and being unflinchingly honest about who you are. It's the quiet confidence that grows from living in alignment with your values, regardless of external pressures or societal expectations.

This power isn't measured by what you own but by who you are when you are alone. It's the ability to remain kind, compassionate, and faithful to yourself, even in adversity. Real power is rooted in love:

- Love for yourself
- Love for those around you
- Love for the ongoing journey of self-discovery and growth

This kind of power drives you to level up, letting you own your strengths and your flaws like the boss you are.

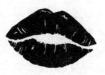

THANK YOU

"**SITTING WITH MY** thoughts and experiences and understanding my emotions throughout writing this book gave me a power I would have never thought I had the ability to access. I cried in therapy sessions, opened up old wounds, strengthened old relationships, and found peace in closing unhealthy relationships. I also learned there is power in knowing that I don't know everything; however, my eyes, ears, and heart are open to learning, being corrected, and navigating what life has to offer." —Mandii

"**WHEN CHARLAMAGNE APPROACHED** us to do this book, I honestly thought I would be writing to a bunch of people that were horny and needed to scratch that itch. I didn't think for a second I would go from telling threesome stories to painful memories that I had to build myself back from. There are moments I can't believe I shared with you, and even though I thought about hitting backspace on a few paragraphs, this was the entire point. The actual purpose of this project was greater than my initial idea. I didn't know that we'd get this deep. But now I see that I needed to be *with* you so this book could be *for* you." —Weezy

NOTES

HOW CAN I EXPECT YOU TO PLEASE ME IF I CAN'T PLEASE MYSELF?

1. Sigmund Freud, *Three Essays on the Theory of Sexuality*, trans. James Strachey (New York: Basic Books, 2000), 125.

2. bell hooks, *Feminism Is for Everybody: Passionate Politics* (Cambridge, MA: South End Press, 2000), 95.

3. Kate Williams, "45 Orgasms Statistics," PleasureBetter.com, November 19, 2024, https://pleasurebetter.com/orgasm-statistics/.

4. Amy Lang, "What's Typical About Youth Sexuality, What's Not, How to Know the Difference," *Youth Today*, February 17, 2020, https://youthtoday.org/2020/02/whats-typical-about-youth-sexuality-whats-not-how-to-know-the-difference/.

5. Robin Hilmantel, "Were You Over or Under the Average Age That Women First Orgasm When It Happened to You?," *Women's Health Magazine*, May 21, 2015, https://www.womenshealthmag.com/sex-and-love/a19923422/when-women-first-orgasm/.

WHY DON'T WE CHEAT TOGETHER?

1. Russell Brand, Goodreads Quotes, https://www.goodreads.com/author/quotes/884168.Russell_Brand.

2. *Sex and the City*, season 1, episode 8, "Three's a Crowd," written by Jenny Bicks, directed by Nicole Holofcener, aired July 26, 1998, on HBO.

3. Robert Weiss, "Why People Cheat on Partners They Still Love," *Psychology Today*, February 23, 2022, https://www.psychologytoday.com/us/blog/love-and-sex-in-the-digital-age/202202/why-people-cheat-on-partners-they-still-love.

4. Esther Perel, *Mating in Captivity: Unlocking Erotic Intelligence* (New York: Harper Perennial, 2006), 36.

DID YOU KNOW YOU CAN FIND UNICORNS IN MEXICO?

1. Ernest Jones, *The Life and Work of Sigmund Freud*, vol. 2 (London: Hogarth Press, 1955), 421.

2. Audre Lorde, *Sister Outsider: Essays and Speeches* (Berkeley, CA: Crossing Press, 1984), 64.

ARE SCISSORS ONLY FOR ARTS AND CRAFTS?

1. Pat Robertson, quoted in Heather Rhoads, "'RACIST, SEXIST, ANTI-GAY': How the Religious Right Helped Defeat Iowa's ERA," *On the Issues Magazine*, 1993, https://ontheissuesmagazine.com/activism/racist-sexist-anti-gay-how-the-religious-right-helped-defeat-iowas-era/.

2. Demi Burnett (@demi_burnett), "So fucking sick of ppl speaking their opinion on my sexuality. I have the freedom to like who I like. If I like a guy, that doesn't mean I'm straight. If I like a girl, that doesn't mean I'm a lesbian. Just let me be and let me love who I want to without trying to categorize me," Twitter (now X), July 21, 2020, https://x.com/demi_burnett/status/1285792411818455046.

3. Kinsey Institute, "Kinsey Scale," accessed December 13, 2024, https://kinseyinstitute.org/research/publications/kinsey-scale.php.

4. WebMD Editorial Contributor, "What Is Scissoring?," WebMD, July 2, 2023, https://www.webmd.com/sex/what-is-scissoring.

CAN I PUT IT BACK THERE?

1. DaBaby, remarks at Rolling Loud Music Festival, Main Stage, July 25, 2021, quoted in Grant Rindner, "How DaBaby's Homophobic Comments at Rolling Loud Set Off a Firestorm," *GQ*, July 29, 2021, https://www.gq.com/story/dababy-rolling-loud-controversy-explained.

2. Caitlin Moran, interview with BBC News, "Caitlin Moran on Female Sexuality and Comedy," *BBC News*, July 3, 2014, https://www.bbc.com/news/entertainment-arts-28141547.

3. Lynne d Johnson, quoted in "Religion and Coming Out Issues for African Americans," Human Rights Campaign Foundation, https://www.hrc.org/resources/religion-and-coming-out-issues-for-african-americans.

4. Michael J. Mishak, "12 States, Including Florida, Still Ban Sodomy a Decade After U.S. Supreme Court Ruling," *The Florida Times-Union*, April 21, 2014, accessed December 13, 2024, https://www.jacksonville.com/story/news/nation-world/2014/04/21/12-states-including-florida-still-ban-sodomy-decade-after-us-supreme/15797271007/.

5. Lisa M. Diamond, Janna A. Dickenson, and Karen L. Blair, "Stability of Sexual Attractions Across Different Timescales: The Roles of Bisexuality and Gender," *Archives of Sexual Behavior* 46, no. 1 (2017): 193–204, https://doi.org/10.1007/s10508-016-0860-x.

6. Centers for Disease Control and Prevention, *Youth Risk Behavior Surveillance—United States, 2019 (Morbidity and Mortality Weekly Report)*, 2020, https://www.cdc.gov/healthyyouth/data/yrbs/pdf/2019/su6901-H.pdf.

7. Alex Hall, quoted in Gabrielle Kassel, "What Goes In Does Come Out—So Here's What You Need to Know About Eating Before Anal Sex," Well+Good, June 3, 2023, https://www.wellandgood.com/eating-before-anal-sex/.

8. Kendall, "Do you have to use an enema or anal douche before you have anal sex?," Planned Parenthood, April 14, 2023, https://www

.plannedparenthood.org/blog/do-you-have-to-use-an-enema-or
-anal-douche-before-you-have-anal-sex.

IS PROTECTION EVEN PLEASURABLE?

1. Oscar Wilde, *Lord Arthur Savile's Crime and Other Stories* (London: James R. Osgood, McIlvaine and Co., 1891), 78.
2. Eleanor Roosevelt, "Thoughts on the Business of Life," Forbes Quotes, https://www.forbes.com/quotes/2610/.
3. Cleveland Clinic, "Bacterial Vaginosis," last modified on December 6, 2023, accessed on December 13, 2024, https://my.clevelandclinic.org /health/diseases/3963-bacterial-vaginosis.

CAN I PUT YOUR PENIS IN A CAGE?

1. Confucius, quoted in Hui Huang, "Do Not Cry for Me, Confucius: The Reconstruction of Chinese Female Identity During the Cultural Revolution," UCLA: Center for the Study of Women, 2010, 1.
2. Donna Summer, "My Fetishes, Continued: Donna Summer," *Penthouse*, July 1979, accessed via https://prince.org/msg/8/284796.
3. Robabeh Potki, Tayebe Ziaei, Mahbobeh Faramarzi, Mahmood Moosazadeh, and Zoreh Shahhosseini, "Bio-Psycho-Social Factors Affecting Sexual Self-Concept: A Systematic Review," *Electronic Physician* 9, no. 9 (2017): 5172–78, https://doi.org/10.19082/5172.

WHY STAND UP WHEN YOU CAN BE ON YOUR KNEES?

1. Wayne A. Mack, *Strengthening Your Marriage* (Phillipsburg, NJ: Presbyterian and Reformed Publishing, 1977), 14.
2. Betty Friedan, *The Feminine Mystique* (New York: W. W. Norton, 1963), 55.
3. Wilbert L. Cooper, "The Sisterhood Behind the Raciest, Rawest Podcast on the Internet," *Vice*, May 7, 2018, https://www.vice.com/en /article/the-sisterhood-behind-the-raciest-rawest-podcast-on -the-internet-whoreible-decisions/.

4. "Submission," Encyclopedia.com, accessed on December 13, 2024, https://www.encyclopedia.com/humanities/dictionaries-thesauruses -pictures-and-press-releases/submission.

WHY DON'T THEY JUST CALL IT A VACUUM?*

1. Friedrich Nietzsche, *Thus Spoke Zarathustra*, trans. Walter Kaufmann (New York: Penguin Books, 1978), 66.
2. Tracee Ellis Ross, *Glamour*'s 2017 Women of the Year Summit speech, Brooklyn, New York City, November 13, 2017, https://www .glamour.com/story/tracee-ellis-ross-glamour-women-of-the-year -speech-2017.
3. Katherine Kortsmit, Antoinette T. Nguyen, Michele G. Mandel, Lisa M. Hollier, Stephanie Ramer, Jessica Rodenhizer, and Maura K. Whiteman, "Abortion Surveillance—United States, 2021," CDC *Morbidity and Mortality Weekly Report* 72, no. 9 (2023): 1–29, https:// www.cdc.gov/mmwr/volumes/72/ss/ss7209a1.htm.
4. Ibid.

WHEN DO YOU KNOW YOU'VE STAYED TOO LONG?

1. Thomas Hardy, *Far from the Madding Crowd* (London: Vintage Books, 2010), 205.
2. Toni Morrison, *Song of Solomon* (New York: Plume, 1987), 306.

WELL, WHAT WERE YOU WEARING?*

1. bell hooks, *Communion: The Female Search for Love* (New York: William Morrow Paperback, 2002), 89.
2. CDC, "Sexual Violence Prevention," January 23, 2024, https://www .cdc.gov/sexual-violence/about/index.html.
3. National Organization for Women, "Black Women and Sexual Violence," 2018, https://now.org/wp-content/uploads/2018/02/Black -Women-and-Sexual-Violence-6.pdf.
4. Amy Novotney, "Women Who Experience Trauma Are Twice as

Likely as Men to Develop PTSD. Here's Why," American Psychological Association, last updated July 8, 2024, https://www.apa.org/topics
/women-girls/women-trauma.

5. Kelly Cue Davis, Cynthia A. Stappenbeck, N. Tatiana Masters, and
William H. George, "Young Women's Experiences with Coercive and
Noncoercive Condom Use Resistance: Examination of an Understud-
ied Sexual Risk Behavior," *Women's Health Issues* 29, no. 3 (May–June
2019), https://www.whijournal.com/article/S1049-3867(18)30334-7
/abstract.

6. Matthew Robinson, "Police Officer Found Guilty of Condom 'Stealthing' in Landmark Trial," CNN, December 20, 2018, https://edition.cnn
.com/2018/12/20/health/stealthing-germany-sexual-assault-scli-intl
/index.html.

7. Sara M. Moniuszko, "What Would a 'Stealthing' Ban Mean for Survivors of Sexual Violence?," *USA Today*, September 13, 2022, https://
www.usatoday.com/story/life/health-wellness/2022/09/13/stealth
ing-condom-removal-legal-us/7929661001/?gnt-cfr=1&gca-cat=p.

8. Joe Hernandez, "California Is the 1st State to Ban 'Stealthing,' Non-
consensual Condom Removal," NPR, October 7, 2021, https://www
.npr.org/2021/10/07/1040160313/california-stealthing-nonconsen
sual-condom-removal.

DO YOU REALIZE YOU RAPED ME?*

1. Jane C. Timm, "Trump on Hot Mic: 'When You're a Star . . . You Can
Do Anything' to Women," NBC News, October 7, 2016, https://www
.nbcnews.com/politics/2016-election/trump-hot-mic-when-you-re
-star-you-can-do-n662116.

2. Margaret Atwood, *The Handmaid's Tale* (New York: Vintage; 1st Anchor Books edition, 1998), 51.

3. J. Murphy-Oikonen et al., "Unfounded Sexual Assault: Women's Experiences of Not Being Believed by the Police," *Journal of Interpersonal*

Violence 37, nos. 11–12 (June 2022): NP8916–NP8940, https://doi .org/10.1177/0886260520978190.

4. RAINN, "Scope of the Problem: Statistics—How Often Does Sexual Assault Occur in the United States?," https://rainn.org/statistics /scope-problem.

5. Centers for Disease Control and Prevention, "Sexual Violence: Prevention Strategies," last reviewed on February 27, 2023, https://www .cdc.gov/sexual-violence/about/index.html#:~:text=The%20perpetra tor%20of%20sexual%20violence,%2C%20online%2C%20or%20 through%20technology.

6. RAIIN, Campus Sexual Abuse: How to Protect Students and Support Survivors, https://rainn.org/education/safe-students-safe-campuses.

7. National Center on Violence Against Women in the Black Community, "Black Women and Sexual Assault," Statistics on Violence Against Black Women, October 2018, https://nwlc.org/wp-content/uploads/2020/05 /Ujima-Womens-Violence-Stats-v7.4-1_Condencia-Brade.pdf.

WHAT'S YOUR PRICE?

1. Martin Luther, quoted in Peter F. Wiener, *Martin Luther: Hitler's Spiritual Ancestor*, 2nd ed. (Cranford, NJ: Amer Atheist Pr, 1999), 94.

2. Jess Zimmerman, "'Where's My Cut?': On Unpaid Emotional Labor," The Toast, July 13, 2015, https://web.archive.org/web/20231117011048 /https://the-toast.net/2015/07/13/emotional-labor/.

3. Rudyard Kipling, "On the City Wall," *In Black and White*, Volume IV, (New York: Charles Scribner's Sons, 1899), 302.

4. Mike Mariani, "Exchanging Sex for Survival," *The Atlantic*, June 26, 2014, https://www.theatlantic.com/health/archive/2014/06/exchanging -sex-for-survival/371822/.

5. Vera Papisova, "Why 'Survival Sex' Is the Only Option for Some Homeless LGBTQ Kids," *Teen Vogue*, February 26, 2016, https://www.teen vogue.com/story/ali-forney-center-homeless-lgbtq-youth-survival-sex.

WHY GET PURSES WHEN YOU CAN
GET A STOCK PORTFOLIO?

1. Aristotle Onassis, quoted in "Aristotle Onassis," Biography.com, April 7, 2021, https://www.biography.com/celebrities/aristotle-onassis.

2. Tiffany Aliche, *The One Week Budget: Learn to Create Your Money Management System in 7 Days or Less!* (CreateSpace Independent Publishing Platform: 2011), 82.

DO MARRIED MEN REALLY TREAT YOU BETTER?

1. Sriprakash Jaiswal, quoted in Afaq Danish, "Afaq Danish Presents His Own 'Modest Proposal' à la Jonathan Swift in a Satirical Hyperbole Mocking Heartless Attidues Towards Women in India," New Age Islam, January 10, 2013, https://www.newageislam.com/letter-editor/afaq-danish-new-age-islam/afaq-danish-presents-his-own-modest-proposal-à-la-jonathan-swift-satirical-hyperbole-mocking-heartless-attitudes-towards-women-india/d/9944.

2. Brenda Jackson, *Delaney's Desert Sheikh* (New York: Silhouette Books, 2002), 45.

3. Carl Zimmer, "Monogamy and Human Evolution," *New York Times*, August 2, 2013, https://www.nytimes.com/2013/08/02/science/monogamys-boost-to-human-evolution.html.

4. Irene Tsapelas, Helen E. Fisher, and Arthur Aron, "Infidelity: When, Where, Why," *The Dark Side of Close Relationships II* (New York: Routledge, 2010), 175–96.

DOES LOVE SHOW UP WHEN YOU AREN'T LOOKING?*

1. Jean Giraudoux, quoted in "All Women Are Born Evil. Some Just Realize Their Potential Later in Life Than Others," AZ Quotes, https://www.azquotes.com/quote/1041973.

2. Frida Kahlo, quoted in Laura Almeida, "Quotes from Frida Kahlo,"

Denver Art Museum, December 28, 2020, https://www.denverartmu seum.org/en/blog/quotes-frida-kahlo.

WHY DO YOU NEED ME TO NEED YOU?

1. Jean-Jacques Rousseau, *Thoughts of Jean-Jacques Rousseau, Citizen of Geneva* (London: J. DeBrett and R. Baldwin, 1788), 154.
2. Cher, "Mom, I Am Rich Man," full interview with Jane Pauley, *Dateline*, 1996, https://www.youtube.com/watch?v=QxnxBsZYCvg.
3. Peter A. Piccione, "The Status of Women in Ancient Egyptian Society," College of Charleston, 1995, cited in Facts and Details, "Women's Rights in Ancient Egypt: Equality, Contracts, Violence," https://africame.factsanddetails.com/article/entry-1122.html.
4. Suzanne McGee and Heidi Moore, "Women's Rights and Their Money: A Timeline from Cleopatra to Lilly Ledbetter," *The Guardian*, August 11, 2014, https://www.theguardian.com/money/us-money -blog/2014/aug/11/women-rights-money-timeline-history#:~:text =US%2C%201848:%20Married%20Woman's%20Property,if%20 she%20were%20still%20single.
5. Rachel F. Seidman, "Voices of Independence: Four Oral Histories about Building Women's Economic Power," Smithsonian American Women's History Museum, October 25, 2024, https://womenshistory .si.edu/blog/voices-independence-four-oral-histories-about-build ing-womens-economic-power#:~:text=As%20a%20result%20of%20 her,to%20build%20their%20financial%20power.

IF 9 MILLION PEOPLE ARE HERE, WHY DO I FEEL ALONE?*

1. *Sex and the City*, season 6, episode 10, "Boy, Interrupted," written by Cindy Chupack, directed by Timothy Van Patten, aired August 24, 2003, on HBO.

ABOUT THE AUTHORS

MANDII B

Born and raised in Orlando, Florida, Mandii B is a powerhouse of talent, resilience, and entrepreneurial spirit. With a rich cultural background blending Jamaican and American influences, she grew up in a single-parent household, developing a strong sense of determination and independence from an early age. She went on to earn both a bachelor of science in accounting and a bachelor of business administration from Lehman College, paving the way for a successful career in finance. Mandii gained invaluable experience working as a public accountant for a prestigious Big Four firm and a Fortune 500 investment bank, but her true calling lay beyond the corporate world. Driven by her passion for storytelling and self-expression, she left finance behind to carve out her own lane in media and entertainment. Today, she empowers and inspires through her thought-provoking podcasts, produces and develops groundbreaking content behind the scenes, and captivates audiences as a host on networks like MTV, Revolt, and BET. She is the proud mother of an orange tabby cat—and a growing empire of businesses.

WEEZYWTF

Featured in *Newsweek* and *Huffington Post* and still trying to figure out exactly why, the Orlando, Florida, native got her start in entertainment by accident. A Black Jewish thirty-something-year-old, WeezyWTF grew up with a passion for life, travel, and the dance floor, leading her to the best city in the world, New York. After starting in corporate tech sales, she figured out quickly that her place wasn't behind a desk. When her dating app sexcapades inspired the renowned *WHOREible Decisions* podcast, her vibrant personality took her further than expected. Weezy is now the owner of WTFMedia Studios located on both coasts, host of the TV show *$ex Sells*, and Head of Podcast Development for Kenya Barris. In her free time, Weezy enjoys spending time with her puppy, Nina, visiting family, and exploring new countries.

TEMPEST X

Tempest X is an author based in Newark, New Jersey, with roots in Reading, Pennsylvania. Of Black, Cherokee, German, and Irish descent, her multicultural heritage deeply informs her work, which often examines American history and Critical Race Theory. A former music executive and jazz singer, Tempest has a natural affinity for music-based projects but prefers to let her imagination—and the whispers of her ancestors—guide her creativity. As she says, "Boxes are boring." Specializing in screenplays, fiction, nonfiction, content adaptation, and memoirs, Tempest thanks Mandii and Weezy for inviting her to join them on this unforgettable book-writing journey.